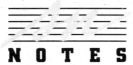

SPRINGHOUSE

N O T E S

MATERNAL NEWBORN NURSING

Lynne Hutnik Conrad, RNC, MSN

Ms. Conrad, the author of this book, is a Nursing Instructor at Holy Family College, Philadelphia. She earned her BSN from Trenton (N.J.) State College, and received her MSN from Villanova (Pa.) University. Ms. Conrad is a member of Sigma Theta Tau, Phi Kappa Phi, National League for Nursing, the Pennsylvania Nurses' Association, and the Nurses' Association of the American College of Obstetricians and Gynecologists.

Linda Phillips Brown, RN, PhD

Dr. Brown, the reviewer of this book, is an Assistant Professor of Nursing at the University of Pennsylvania, Philadelphia. She earned her BSN from Temple University, Philadelphia, and received her MSN and PhD from the University of Pennsylvania. Dr. Brown is a member of Sigma Theta Tau.

Springhouse Publishing Company
Springhouse, Pennsylvania

STAFF FOR THIS VOLUME

CLINICAL STAFF

Clinical Director
Barbara McVan, RN

Clinical Editors
Lynne Atkinson, RN, BSN, CEN
Joan E. Mason, RN, EdM
Diane Schweisguth, RN, BSN, CCRN, CEN

ADVISORY BOARD

Mildred Wernet Boyd, RN, BSN, MSN
Assistant Professor, Essex Community College,
Baltimore

Dorothy Brooten, PhD, FAAN
Chairperson, Health Care of Women and
Childbearing Section, Director of Graduate Perinatal
Nursing, University of Pennsylvania School of
Nursing, Philadelphia

Lillian S. Brunner, MSN, ScD, LittD, FAAN
Nurse/Author, Brunner Associates, Inc., Berwyn, Pa.

Irma J. D'Antonio, RN, PhD
Professor and Chairperson, Department of Nursing,
Mount St. Mary's College, Los Angeles

Kathleen Dracup, RN, DNSc, FAAN
Associate Professor, School of Nursing, University of
California, Los Angeles, Los Angeles

Cecile A. Lengacher, RN, PhD
Director of the Division of Nursing and Health
Sciences, Manatee Junior College, Bradenton, Fla.

Barbara Tower, RN, MSN, CCRN
Assistant Professor, Essex Community College,
Baltimore

PUBLICATION STAFF

Executive Director, Editorial
Stanley Loeb

Executive Director, Creative Services
Jean Robinson

Design
John Hubbard (art director), Stephanie Peters
(associate art director), Jacalyn Bove Facciolo,
Julie Carleton Barlow, Darcey Feralio

Editing
Donna L. Hilton (acquisitions), Kathy E. Goldberg,
Patricia McKeown, David Prout

Copy Editing
David Moreau (manager), Edith McMahon
(supervisor), Nick Anastasio, Keith de Pinho, Diane
Labus, Doris Weinstock, Debra Young

Art Production
Robert Perry (manager), Anna Brindisi, Christopher
Buckley, Loretta Caruso, Donald Knauss, Christina
McKinley, Mark Marcin, Robert Wieder

Typography
David Kosten (manager), Diane Paluba (assistant
manager), Joyce Rossi Biletz, Alicia Dempsey,
Brenda Mayer, Nancy Wirs

Manufacturing
Deborah Meiris (manager)

Project Coordination
Aline S. Miller (supervisor), Maureen Carmichael

Library of Congress Cataloging-in-Publication Data

Conrad, Lynne H.
  Maternal—newborn nursing.

  (Springhouse notes)
  Includes bibliographies and index.
    1. Obstetrical nursing. 2. Infants (Newborn)—
Diseases—Nursing. I. Title. II. Series. [DNLM:
1. Neonatology—nurses' instruction.
  2. Obstetrical Nursing.   WY 157.3 C754m]
RG951.C67   1988   610.73'678   87-26743
ISBN 0-87434-111-6

Contents

How to Use Springhouse Notes

Today, more than ever, nursing students face enormous time pressures. Nursing education has become more sophisticated, increasing the difficulties students have with studying efficiently and keeping pace.

The need for a comprehensive, well-designed series of study aids is great, which is why we've produced Springhouse Notes...to meet that need. Springhouse Notes provide essential course material in outline form, enabling the nursing student to study more effectively, improve understanding, achieve higher test scores, and get better grades.

Key features appear throughout each book, making the information more accessible and easier to remember.
- **Learning Objectives.** These objectives precede each section in the book to help the student evaluate knowledge before and after study.
- **Key Points.** Highlighted in color throughout the book, these points provide a way to quickly review critical information. Key points may include:
  —a cardinal sign or symptom of a disorder
  —the most current or popular theory about a topic
  —a distinguishing characteristic of a disorder
  —the most important step of a process
  —a critical assessment component
  —a crucial nursing intervention
  —the most widely used or successful therapy or treatment.
- **Points to Remember.** This information, found at the end of each section, summarizes the section in capsule form.
- **Glossary.** Difficult, frequently used, or sometimes misunderstood terms are defined for the student at the end of each section.

Remember: Springhouse Notes are learning tools designed to *help* you. They are not intended for use as a primary information source. They should never substitute for class attendance, text reading, or classroom note taking.

This book, Maternal-Newborn Nursing, begins with the structure and function of male and female reproductive organs. Next, all the details you'll need to remember—from intrauterine development through the postpartum period and the normal newborn—are presented. Also discussed are characteristics, assessment, and care of the normal and high-risk newborn and assessment and management of a high-risk pregnancy. The definition, pathophysiology, clinical manifestations, management, and (where appropriate) fetal and maternal implications are given for each disorder covered. Nursing roles, responsibilities, and interventions are discussed throughout.

Structure and Function of Reproductive Organs

Learning Objectives

After studying this section, the reader should be able to:

- Describe the structure and functions of the male and female reproductive organs.

- Describe the function that secretions from the accessory sex glands perform in the reproductive cycle.

- Identify the function of the male and female organs within the reproductive process.

- Describe the hormonal and uterine changes that occur during the menstrual cycle.

I. Structure and Function of the Reproductive Organs

A. **Male reproductive system: external genitals**
  1. Penis: three layers of erectile tissue; two corpora cavernosa and one corpus spongiosum
     a. Consists of the body (shaft) and glans
     b. Deposits sperm in the female reproductive tract
  2. Scrotum: pouchlike structure composed of skin, fascial connective tissue, and smooth muscle fibers
     a. Contains two lateral compartments, which house the testes and related structures
     b. Protects the testes and sperm from high body temperature

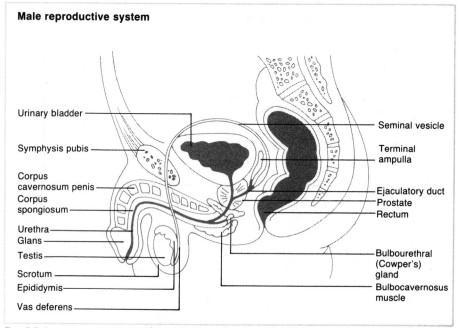

Male reproductive system

B. **Male reproductive system: internal genitals**
  1. Testes: Two oval-shaped glandular organs inside the scrotum
     a. Site of sperm and androgen production
     b. Site of testosterone production, the primary male sex hormone
  2. Epididymides: Initial section of the testes' excretory duct system
     a. Stores sperm as they mature and become motile
     b. Produces some seminal fluid
  3. Vas deferens: a connection between the epididymal lumen and the prostatic urethra; a conduit for sperm
  4. Ejaculatory ducts: a passageway for semen and fluid secreted by the seminal vesicles

5. Urethra: a passageway for urine and semen; it runs through the penis from the bladder to the external urethral opening

C. **Male accessory glands**
1. Seminal vesicles: two pouchlike structures
   a. Located between the bladder and rectum
   b. Secrete a viscous fluid that aids in sperm motility and metabolism
2. Prostate gland: glandular and muscular tissue
   a. Located just below the bladder
   b. Considered the homologue of the female Skene's glands
   c. The urethra runs through the center of the prostate
   d. Produces an alkaline fluid that enhances sperm motility and lubricates the urethra during sexual activity
3. Bulbourethral glands (Cowper's glands): two pea-sized glands that open into the posterior portion of the urethra. Secrete a thick alkaline fluid that neutralizes acidic female secretions, thus enhancing sperm survival

D. **Female reproductive system: external genitals**
1. Mons pubis: adipose cushion over the anterior symphysis pubis
   a. Protects the pelvic bones
   b. Adds to sensuality and rounded contour of the female body
2. Labia majora
   a. Consists of connective tissue, elastic fibers, veins, and sebaceous glands
   b. Protects the components of the vulval cleft
3. Labia minora: connective tissue, sebaceous and sweat glands, nonstriated muscle fibers, nerve endings, and blood vessels
   a. The two labia minora unite to form the fourchette
   b. Their secretions lubricate the vulva, add to sexual enjoyment, and provide bactericidal agents
4. Clitoris: erectile tissue, nerves, and blood vessels
   a. Consists of the glans, body, and two crura
   b. Corresponds to the penis
   c. Provides sexual pleasure
5. Vaginal vestibule: tissue extending from the clitoris to the posterior fourchette
   a. The vaginal orifice, hymen, fossa navicularis, and Bartholin's glands compose the vaginal vestibule

    b. The hymen is a thin, vascularized mucous membrane at the vaginal orifice or opening

    c. The fossa navicularis is a depressed area between the hymen and fourchette

    d. The Bartholin's glands are two bean-shaped glands on either side of the vagina; they secrete mucus in response to sexual stimulation

6. Perineal body: the area between the vagina and anus; site of episiotomy during childbirth

7. Urethral meatus: Located 1 to 2.5 cm below the clitoris

8. Paraurethral glands (Skene's glands)

    a. Produce mucus

    b. Located immediately inside the urethral meatus

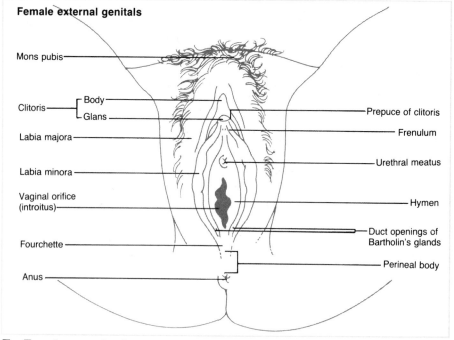

Female external genitals

Mons pubis

Clitoris — Body / Glans

Labia majora

Labia minora

Vaginal orifice (introitus)

Fourchette

Anus

Prepuce of clitoris

Frenulum

Urethral meatus

Hymen

Duct openings of Bartholin's glands

Perineal body

E. Female reproductive system: internal genitals

1. Vagina: vascularized musculomembranous tube

    a. Extends from the external genitals to the uterus

    b. Functions as the copulatory and parturient passage

    c. Acts as an excretory duct of the uterus for menses and other secretions

2. Uterus: a hollow pear-shaped muscular organ divided into an upper (body or corpus) and lower portion (cervix) by a slight constriction (isthmus)

    a. Body or corpus consists of three layers: the perimetrium, the myometrium, and the endometrium

UTeRus -(INvoluntary)you cannoT conTRol ,T.)
SmooTh muscle

    b. Uterus provides an environment for fetal growth and development
    c. Uterus receives support from the broad, round, and uterosacral ligaments
  3. Fallopian tubes
    a. Route of transport of ovum from ovary to uterus; approximately 12 cm long
    b. Site of fertilization; nourishing environment for zygote
    c. Divided into four portions: the interstitial, the isthmus, the ampulla, and the fimbria
    d. Consists of four layers: peritoneal, subserous, muscular, and mucous
  4. Ovaries
    a. Two almond-shaped glandular structures on either side of the uterus, below and behind the fallopian tubes
    b. Site of ovulation and production of steroid sex hormones (estrogens, progesterone, androgens)

Female internal genitals

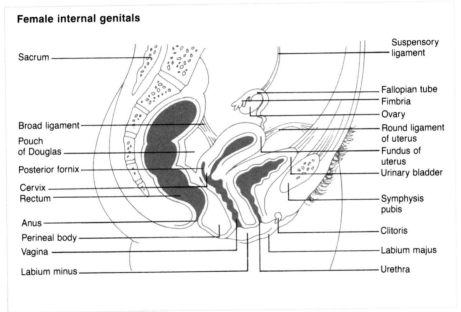

Sacrum

Broad ligament
Pouch of Douglas
Posterior fornix
Cervix
Rectum
Anus
Perineal body
Vagina
Labium minus

Suspensory ligament
Fallopian tube
Fimbria
Ovary
Round ligament of uterus
Fundus of uterus
Urinary bladder
Symphysis pubis
Clitoris
Labium majus
Urethra

F. Female accessory glands
  1. Breasts: glandular, fibrous, and adipose tissue
    a. Grow and develop from stimulation of secretions from the hypothalamus, anterior pituitary, and ovaries
    b. Provide nourishment to infant
    c. Transfer maternal antibodies during breastfeeding
    d. Enhance sexual pleasure

G. Female reproductive cycle
1. Menstrual phase: days 1 through 5 of menstrual cycle
   a. Estrogen and progesterone levels decrease
   b. Elevated levels of follicle-stimulating hormone (FSH) and steady levels of luteinizing hormone (LH) initiate estrogen secretion by the ovary
   c. Menstrual flow begins
2. Proliferative (follicular) phase: days 6 through 14
   a. Increased estrogen production leads to proliferation of endometrium and myometrium in preparation for possible implantation
   b. Follicle secretes estradiol
   c. FSH stimulates graafian follicle
   d. FSH production decreases before ovulation, which occurs at approximately day 14
3. Secretory (luteal) phase: days 15 and 16
   a. Corpus luteum is formed under the influence of LH
   b. Estrogen and progesterone production increases
   c. Endometrium is prepared for implantation of fertilized ovum
4. Ischemic phase: days 27 and 28
   a. The corpus luteum degenerates if conception does not occur
   b. Estrogen and progesterone levels decline if conception does not occur

Points to Remember

The primary male sex hormone is testosterone.

Sperm survival and motility depend upon the alkaline secretions of the accessory sex glands.

The female reproductive cycle is marked by cyclic hormonal changes.

Fertilization occurs within the fallopian tubes.

Glossary

Corpus luteum—the ruptured graafian follicle develops into a yellow structure that secretes progesterone during the second half of the menstrual cycle. If pregnancy occurs, the corpus luteum will continue to produce progesterone until the placenta assumes that function

Follicle-stimulating hormone—hormone produced by the anterior pituitary gland; stimulates the development of the graafian follicle

Luteinizing hormone—hormone produced by the anterior pituitary gland; stimulates ovulation and the development of the corpus luteum

Seminal fluid—male ejaculate containing sperm and secretions from accessory sex glands

Intrauterine Development

Learning Objectives

After studying this section, the reader should be able to:

- Describe the structure and function of the placenta.

- Describe the stages of embryonic and fetal development.

- Describe fetal-placental circulation.

- Describe the composition and functions of the amniotic fluid and umbilical cord.

II. Intrauterine Development

A. Gametogenesis: the production of specialized sex cells (gametes)

1. The male gamete (sperm) is produced in the seminiferous tubules of the testes during spermatogenesis
2. The female gamete (ovum) is produced in the graafian follicle of the ovary during oogenesis
3. The number of chromosomes the gametes contain is halved (meiosis) from 46 to 23 as they mature

B. Conception (fertilization): the fusion of the sperm and ovum (oocyte) in the ampulla of the fallopian tube

1. The fertilized egg is called a zygote
2. The diploid number of chromosomes (44 autosomes and 2 sex chromosomes) is restored when the zygote is formed
3. A male zygote is formed if the ovum is fertilized by a sperm carrying a Y chromosome; if the ovum is fertilized by a sperm carrying an X chromosome, a female zygote results

C. Cellular multiplication

1. The zygote undergoes mitosis, dividing into two cells, four cells, and so on, which are called blastomeres
2. Blastomeres eventually form the morula, a solid ball of cells
3. After the morula enters the uterus, a cavity then forms within the dividing cells, thus changing the morula into a blastocyst

D. Implantation

1. The cellular wall of the blastocyst (the trophoblast) implants itself in the endometrium of the anterior or posterior fundal region 7 to 9 days after fertilization
2. Primary villa appear within weeks after implantation

E. Decidua: after implantation, the endometrium is called the decidua

F. Placentation: the chorionic villi invade the endometrium and become the fetal portion of the future placenta

G. Fetal membranes

1. Chorion: The fetal membrane closest to the uterine wall; it gives rise to the placenta
2. Amnion: The inner fetal membrane that lines the amniotic sac

H. Umbilical cord: the lifeline from the embryo to the placenta
1. Measures approximately 50 to 55 cm in length and 2 cm in diameter at term
2. Contains two arteries and one vein
3. Contains Wharton's jelly, a gelatinous substance that helps prevent kinking of the cord in utero
4. Blood flows through cord at the rate of approx. 400 ml/min

I. Placenta
1. Structure
   a. Contains 15 to 20 subdivisions called cotyledons
   b. Weighs approximately 400 to 600 g (1 to 1.3 lb), measures 15 to 20 cm (6 to 10 inches) in diameter, and is 2.5 to 3 cm (1 inch) thick at term
   c. Feels rough in texture and appears reddish on maternal surface; fetal surface is shiny and grayish
2. Physiology
   a. Placenta functions as a transport mechanism between the mother and fetus
   b. Its life span depends upon oxygen consumption
   c. Placental function depends upon maternal circulation
   d. Circulation to the fetus and placenta is best when the mother lies on her left side
3. Functions
   a. Receives maternal oxygen via diffusion
   b. Produces all hormones except ACTH
   c. Supplies the fetus with carbohydrates, water, fats, protein, minerals, and inorganic salts
   d. Carries end products of fetal metabolism into the maternal circulation for excretion
   e. Transfers passive immunity via maternal antibodies

J. Amniotic fluid
1. The uterus, at term, contains 800 to 1,200 ml of clear yellowish fluid whose specific gravity is 1.007 to 1.025; pH 7.0 to 7.25
2. Amniotic fluid contains albumin, lanugo, urea, creatinine, bilirubin, fat, enzymes, lecithin, sphingomyelin, and leukocytes
3. Amniotic fluid is replaced every 3 hours
4. Maternal serum provides amniotic fluid in early gestation, with increasing amounts derived from fetal urine late in gestation
5. Functions of amniotic fluid are as follows:
   a. Prevents heat loss and preserves constant fetal body temperatures
   b. Cushions the fetus
   c. Acts as an excretion-collection system
   d. Facilitates fetal growth and development

K. Embryonic development and fetal maturation

1. Embryonic organs and tissues arise from three primary germ layers
   a. Ectoderm: epidermis, nervous system pituitary gland, tooth enamel, salivary glands, optic lens, lining of the lower portion of the anal canal, hair
   b. Endoderm: epithelial lining of the larynx, trachea, bladder, urethra, prostate, auditory canal, liver, pancreas, and alimentary canal
   c. Mesoderm: connective and sclerous tissue, blood and vascular system, musculature, teeth (except enamel), mesothelial lining of the pericardial, pleural, and peritoneal cavities, kidneys and ureters

2. Respiratory system

Gestational age	Development
4 to 7 weeks*	• Primary lung, tracheal, and bronchi buds appear • Nasal pits form • Abdominal and thoracic cavities separated by the diaphragm
8 to 12 weeks	• Bronchioles branch • Pleural and pericardial cavities appear • Lungs assume definitive shape
13 to 20 weeks	• Terminal and respiratory bronchioles appear
21 to 28 weeks	• Nostrils open • Surfactant production begins • Respiratory movements possible • Alveolar ducts and sacs appear
38 to 40 weeks	• Pulmonary branching two-thirds complete • Lecithin/sphingomyelin (L/S) ratio 2:1

3. Genitourinary system

Gestational age	Development
4 to 7 weeks	• Rudimentary ureteral buds present
8 to 12 weeks	• Bladder and urethra separate from rectum; bladder expands as a sac • Kidneys can secrete urine
13 to 20 weeks	• Kidneys in proper position with definitive shape
36 weeks	• Formation of new nephrons ceases

*all weeks are approximate

4. Nervous system

Gestational age	Development
4 weeks	• Well-marked midbrain flexure • Neural groove closed • Spinal cord extends the entire length of spine
8 weeks	• Differentiation of cerebral cortex, meninges, ventricular foramens, and cerebral spinal fluid circulation
12 to 16 weeks	• Structural configuration of brain roughly completed • Cerebral lobes delineated • Cerebellum assumes prominence
20 to 24 weeks	• Brain grossly formed • Myelination of spinal cord begins • Spinal cord ends at S-1
28 to 36 weeks	• Cerebral fissures appear • Convolutions appear • Spinal cord ends at L-3
40 weeks	• Myelination of brain has begun

5. Gastrointestinal system

Gestational age	Development
4 weeks	• Oral cavity and primitive jaw present • Stomach, ducts of pancreas, and liver form • Division of esophagus and trachea begins
8 to 11 weeks	• Intestinal villi form • Small intestines coil in umbilical cord
12 to 16 weeks	• Bile is secreted • Intestines withdraw from umbilical cord to normal position • Meconium present in bowel • Anus open
20 weeks	• Enamel/dentin is deposited • Ascending colon appears • Fetus can suck and swallow • Peristaltic movements begin

6. Hepatic system

Gestational age	Development
4 weeks	• Liver function begins
6 weeks	• Hematopoiesis by liver begins

7. Endocrine system

Gestational age	Development
2 to 3 weeks	● Thyroid tissue appears
4 weeks	● Thyroid can synthesize thyroxine
10 weeks	● Islets of Langerhans differentiated
12 weeks	● Thyroid secretes hormones ● Insulin present in pancreas

8. Reproductive system

Gestational age	Development
2 to 3 weeks	● Sex is determined
6 to 8 weeks	● Sex glands appear ● Differentiation of sex glands into ovaries or testes begins ● External genitalia appear similar
12 to 24 weeks	● Testes descend into the inguinal canal ● External genitalia distinguishable

9. Musculoskeletal system

Gestational age	Development
4 weeks	● Limb buds appear
8 weeks	● First identification of ossification (mandible, humerus, occiput)
12 weeks	● Some bones well outlined ● Ossification continues
16 weeks	● Joint cavities present ● Muscular movements detectable
20 weeks	● Ossification of sternum ● Mother can detect fetal movements (quickening)
28 to 32 weeks	● Ossification continues ● Fetus can turn head to side
36 weeks	● Muscle tone developed; fetus can turn and elevate head

10. Cardiovascular system

Gestational age	Development
2 to 4 weeks	• Heart begins to form • Blood circulation begins • Primitive RBCs circulate • Tubular heart beat by 24 days
5 to 7 weeks	• Atrial division • Heart chambers present • Fetal heart beat detectable • Groups of blood cells identifiable
8 weeks	• Development of heart complete • Fetal circulation follows two circuits; two intraembryonic and four extraembryonic circuits
16 to 20 weeks	• Fetal heart tones audible with fetoscope

11. Fetal circulation: five structures differentiate fetal from extrauterine circulation (see chart p. 19)
    a. Umbilical vein: carries oxygenated blood to the fetus from the placenta
    b. Umbilical arteries: carry deoxygenated blood from the fetus back to the placenta
    c. Foramen ovale: septal opening between the atria of the fetal heart
    d. Ductus arteriosus: connection between the pulmonary artery and aorta that allows shunting of blood around the fetal lungs
    e. Ductus venosus: carries oxygenated blood from the umbilical vein to the inferior vena cava, bypassing the liver

12. Weight and crown-to-rump measurements

Gestational age	Weight	Crown-to-rump
4 weeks	0.4 g	0.4–0.5 cm
8 weeks	2 g	2.5–3.0 cm
12 weeks	19 g	6.0–9.0 cm
16 weeks	100 g	11.5–13.5 cm
20 weeks	300 g	16.0–18.5 cm
24 weeks	600 g	23 cm
28 weeks	1,100 g	27 cm
32 weeks	1,800–2,100 g	31 cm
36 weeks	2,200–2,900 g	35 cm
40 weeks	3,200+ g	40 cm

FETAL CIRCULATION

The charts below illustrate fetal blood flow. The first chart shows the flow of blood from the placenta to the inferior vena cava. Once the blood reaches the inferior vena cava, the majority of blood flows back to the placenta as shown in the second chart. However, a small amount of blood flows differently, as shown in the third chart.

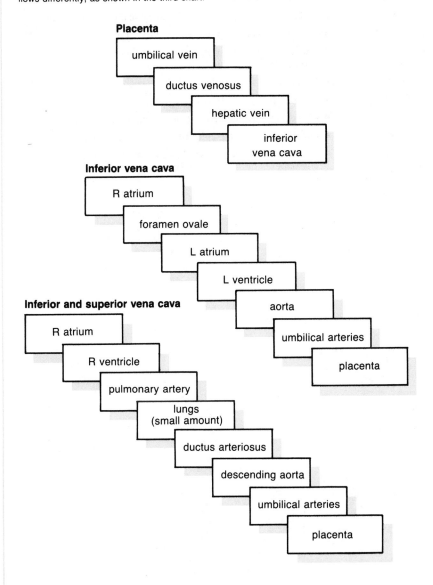

Placenta

umbilical vein

ductus venosus

hepatic vein

inferior vena cava

Inferior vena cava

R atrium

foramen ovale

L atrium

L ventricle

aorta

umbilical arteries

placenta

Inferior and superior vena cava

R atrium

R ventricle

pulmonary artery

lungs (small amount)

ductus arteriosus

descending aorta

umbilical arteries

placenta

13. External appearance

Gestational age	Development
4 weeks	• C-shaped body; pigment in eyes; auditory pit enclosed
8 weeks	• Flat nose, eyes far apart; digits well formed; recognizable eyes, ears, nose, and mouth
12 weeks	• Nails appear; pink, delicate skin, lacrimal ducts developing
16 weeks	• Dominant head; scalp hair present; sweat glands developing
20 weeks	• Vernix, lanugo, and sebaceous glands appear; legs considerably lengthened
24 weeks	• Skin red and wrinkled; eyes structurally complete
28 weeks	• Eyelids open
32 weeks	• Increasing amount of subcutaneous fat; pink, smooth skin
36 weeks	• Lanugo disappearing; soft earlobes with little cartilage
40 weeks	• Copious vernix; moderate to profuse hair; lanugo on shoulders and upper body; ear lobes stiffer with cartilage

Points to Remember

All embryonic tissues and organs are derived from one of the three primary germ layers: the ectoderm, endoderm, and mesoderm.

The umbilical cord is the fetus' lifeline to its mother.

Embryonic maturation follows a distinct pattern, though exact timing of development may differ.

The five structures that differentiate fetal circulation from extrauterine circulation are the ductus venosus, ductus arteriosus, foramen ovale, and the umbilical vein and arteries.

Glossary

Cotyledon—one of the rounded segments on the maternal side of the placenta, consisting of villi, fetal vessels, and an intervillous space

Embryo—conceptus from time of implantation to 5 to 8 weeks

Fetus—conceptus from 5 to 8 weeks until term

Ovum—conceptus from time of conception until primary villi appear; approximately 4 weeks after the last menstrual period

Genetics

Learning Objectives

After studying this section, the reader should be able to:

- Describe basic principles of genetics.

- Describe common genetic disorders.

- Identify clients who require genetic counseling, screening, and testing.

- Discuss common screening and diagnostic techniques.

- Describe the nurse's role in caring for the family with a possible genetic disorder.

- Identify normal reactions of parents after the diagnosis of a genetic disorder.

III. Genetics

A. Basic concepts

1. Genetic information is stored on tightly coiled strands of deoxyribonucleic acid (DNA), called chromosomes
2. Chromosomes are composed of DNA, histone proteins, and nonhistone proteins
3. Chromosomes contain thousands of genes, which are the smallest units of hereditary information, lined up in a specific pattern
4. The normal number of chromosomes is 46: 22 pairs of autosomes and one pair of sex chromosomes (X for female and Y for male)
5. A pictorial analysis of chromosomes (karotype) can be performed most easily on lymphocytes, but also on skin, bone marrow, or organ tissue
6. A genetic disorder can be classified as either congenital or hereditary in nature

B. Mendel's laws

1. Principle of dominance
    a. Genes are not equal in strength
    b. The stronger gene, which produces an observable trait, is called dominant
    c. The weaker gene, whose trait is not seen, is called recessive
2. Principle of segregation
    a. The paired chromosomes that contain genes from both parents separate during meiosis
    b. Chance determines whether the maternal or paternal gene travels to a specific gamete
3. Principle of independent assortment: the pair of one set of genes are distributed in the gametes in random fashion unrelated to any other pairs

C. Categories of genetic disorders

1. Single gene
    a. Traits are determined by two genes, one from each parent
    b. Autosomal traits are determined by a gene on an autosome
    c. Sex-linked traits are determined by a gene on a sex chromosome
    d. The disease trait in autosomal-dominant inheritance disorders is heterozygous and the disorders are due to an abnormal dominant gene on an autosome. Examples include Marfan's syndrome, osteogenesis imperfecta, and Huntington's chorea.
    e. The disease trait in autosomal-recessive inheritance disorders is homozygous. Because the normal gene is dominant, the individual must have two abnormal genes to be affected. Examples include sickle cell anemia, Tay-Sachs disease, cystic fibrosis, and most metabolic diseases.

      f. The abnormal gene in X-linked recessive inheritance disorders is carried on the X chromosome. Examples include hemophilia, Duchenne muscular dystrophy, and color blindness.

      g. X-linked dominant inheritance disorders are similar to X-linked recessive, except that heterozygous females are affected. They are rare. Examples include vitamin D-resistant rickets.

  2. Chromosomal aberrations: deviations in either the number or structure of chromosomes

      a. A structural defect can be due to a loss, addition, or rearrangement of the genes on a chromosome or the exchange of genes between chromosomes

      b. Deviations in the number of chromosomes involve either the gain or loss of an entire chromosome during cell division. The suffix "-somy" is used in disorders with abnormal numbers.

      c. Nondisjunction is the failure of chromosomes to separate during cell division

      d. Translocation is the joining together of two chromosomes to make one large double chromosome.

      e. The most common chromosomal disorder is Down's syndrome (trisomy 21)

  3. Multifactorial inheritance disorders

      a. Disorders in which genes and the environment interact to produce an aberration

      b. Disorders in which no inheritance pattern is identifiable, but where a higher risk of recurrence is observed in certain families

      c. Such disorders include cleft lip and palate, congenital dislocated hip, congenital heart defects, neural tube defects, and pyloric stenosis

D. Detection of genetic disorders

  1. Preconception: indications

      a. For members of a high-risk group (e.g., Tay-Sachs disease among Ashkenazic Jews)

      b. For members of families with a history of genetic disorder(s)

  2. Prenatal testing: indications

      a. A woman age 40 or older

      b. A couple that has previously produced a child with a genetic disorder

      c. A couple that is heterozygous for a recessive disorder

      d. A couple where one or both partners have a genetic disorder

      e. A mother who is a carrier of an X-linked disorder

  3. Prenatal testing: methods

      a. Amniocentesis

      b. Ultrasonography: detects anencephaly, microcephaly, and hydrocephaly

      c. Roentgenography: detects bone abnormalities

4. Postdelivery detection
   a. Biochemical tests for PKU, hypothyroidism, and galactosemia
   b. Cytologic studies for infants whose appearances suggest a chromosomal aberration
   c. Dermatoglyphics to determine chromosomal aberrations through the evaluation of dermal ridges

E. Role of the nurse
1. Understand genetic theory well enough to reinforce information given by the genetic counselor
2. Prepare clients for diagnostic tests by explaining the purpose and procedure of each test
3. Assist with diagnostic testing as necessary
4. Provide emotional support throughout the counseling process
5. Act as an advocate/counselor and teacher
6. Anticipate common responses to diagnoses of genetic disorders, such as apathy, denial, anger, hostility, fear, embarrassment, grief, and decreased self-esteem

Points to Remember

All individual biological and behavioral characteristics are dictated by hereditary material, called genes.

Pregnancies in which a fetus may be affected by a genetic disorder must be individually evaluated.

To provide comprehensive nursing care, the nurse must understand basic genetic concepts.

The occurrence of a genetic disorder can produce a multitude of reactions within the family.

Glossary

Aberration—a deviation from what is typical or normal

Congenital disorder—one that is present at birth and may be due to genetic and/or environmental factors

Hereditary disease—one that is passed from one generation to another

Mutation—a change in a gene or chromosome in gametes

The Prenatal Period

Learning Objectives

After studying this section, the reader should be able to:

- Describe the physiologic and psychological adaptations to pregnancy

- Explain causes of and interventions for common discomforts of pregnancy

- Describe potential complications of pregnancy

- Describe the nutritional needs of the pregnant woman

- Describe common methods of assessing fetal status

- Identify major points to include when counseling a pregnant woman

IV. The Prenatal Period

A. Signs and symptoms of pregnancy

1. Presumptive
   a. Amenorrhea in approximately 80% of women; 20% have slight, painless spotting of unknown cause in early gestation
   b. Nausea and vomiting occurring at any time
   c. Urinary frequency and urgency
   d. Enlarged, tender breasts
   e. Fatigue
   f. Quickening
   g. Thinning and softening of fingernails
   h. Increased skin pigmentation
2. Probable
   a. Uterine enlargement
   b. Goodell's sign: softening of the cervix
   c. Chadwick's sign: bluish mucous membranes of the vagina, cervix, and vulva
   d. Hegar's sign: softening of the lower uterine segment
   e. Braxton-Hicks contractions: painless contractions of the uterus that occur throughout pregnancy
   f. Ballottement: passive fetal movement in response to tapping of the lower portion of the uterus/cervix
   g. Positive pregnancy test results
3. Positive
   a. Fetal heartbeat detected by 17 to 20 weeks of gestation
   b. Ultrasonography results as early as 6 weeks of gestation
   c. Fetal movements felt by examiner

B. Physiologic adaptations to pregnancy

1. Cardiovascular system
   a. Cardiac hypertrophy, due to increased blood volume and cardiac output
   b. Elevation of the heart upward and to the left, due to displacement of the diaphragm
   c. Progressive blood volume increase, peaking in the third trimester at 30 to 50% of prepregnancy levels
   d. Varying resting pulse rate, with increases ranging from 0 to 15 beats/min at term
   e. Pulmonic systolic and apical systolic murmurs, due to decreased blood viscosity and increased blood flow
   f. Increased femoral venous pressure, due to retarded circulation from lower extremities as a result of pressure from enlarged uterus on the pelvic veins and inferior vena cava
   g. Decreased cerebral spinal fluid space, due to enlargement of vessels surrounding the spinal cord dura mater

    h. Increased fibrinogen levels (up to 50% at term) due to hormonal influences

    i. Increased levels of blood coagulation factors VII, IX, and X, leading to a hypercoagulate state

    j. Total red blood cell volume increased by approximately 33%, despite hemodilution and decreased erythrocyte count

    k. Hematocrit decreased by approximately 7%

    l. Total hemoglobin increased by 12 to 15%. This is less than the overall plasma volume increase, thus reducing hemoglobin concentration and leading to physiologic anemia of pregnancy

    m. Leukocyte production equal to or slightly greater than blood volume increase; average leukocyte count is 10,000 to 11,000/mm; peaking at 25,000/mm during labor, possibly through an estrogen-related mechanism

2. Gastrointestinal system

    a. Swelling of gums from increased levels of estrogen; gums may be spongy and hyperemic

    b. Lateral and posterior displacement of intestines

    c. Superior and lateral displacement of the stomach

    d. Delayed intestinal motility and gastric and gallbladder emptying time from smooth muscle relaxation caused by high levels of placental progesterone

    e. Hemorrhoids in later pregnancy from venous pressure

    f. Constipation from increased progesterone levels, resulting in increased water absorption from the colon

    g. Displacement of the appendix away from McBurney's point, making diagnosis of appendicitis difficult

3. Endocrine system

    a. Basal metabolic rate increased by 25% at term from demands of the fetus and uterus and from increased oxygen consumption

    b. Slight hyperplasia of the thyroid due to estrogen levels, resulting in increased iodine metabolism

    c. Slight parathyroidism in response to increased requirement for calcium and vitamin D

    d. Elevated plasma parathormone levels, peaking between 15 and 35 weeks of gestation

    e. Slightly enlarged pituitary gland

    f. Increased production of prolactin by pituitary gland

    g. Increased estrogen levels and hypertrophy of adrenal cortex

    h. Increased cortisol levels, which regulate protein and carbohydrate metabolism

    i. Decreased maternal blood glucose levels

    j. Decreased production of insulin in early pregnancy

    k. Increased production of estrogen, progesterone, and human chorionic somatomammotrophin (HCS) by the placenta and increased levels of maternal cortisol reduce mother's ability to use insulin, thus ensuring an adequate glucose supply for the fetus and placenta

4. Respiratory system
   a. Increased vascularization of the respiratory tract from estrogen
   b. Shortening of the lungs from enlarging uterus
   c. Upward displacement of the diaphragm by the uterus
   d. Increased tidal volume, causing slight hyperventilation
   e. Chest circumference increased by approximately 6 cm
   f. Abdominal breathing replaced by thoracic breathing as pregnancy progresses
   g. Slight increase (two breaths/min) in respiratory rate
   h. Lowered threshold for CO_2 from estrogen and progesterone

5. Metabolic system
   a. Increased water retention due to increased levels of steroidal sex hormones, decreased serum protein levels, and increased intracapillary pressure and permeability
   b. Increased serum lipids, lipoproteins, and cholesterol
   c. Increased iron requirements from fetal demands
   d. Increased carbohydrate needs
   e. Increased protein retention for hyperplasia and hypertrophy of maternal tissues
   f. Weight gain from 25 to 30 lbs; can be divided into 3-, 12-, and 12-lb increments in 1st, 2nd, and 3rd trimesters respectively
   g. Weight gain caused by fetus (7.5 lbs), placenta, and membranes (1.5 lbs), amniotic fluid (2 lbs), uterus (2.5 lbs), breasts (3 lbs), blood volume (2 to 4 lbs), and extravascular fluid and fat reserves (4 to 9 lbs)

6. Integumentary system
   a. Pigmentary changes from increase of melanocyte-stimulating hormone, which results from increased estrogen and progesterone
   b. Hyperactive sweat and sebaceous glands
   c. Darkening of nipples, areola, cervix, vagina, and vulva
   d. Pigmentary changes on the nose, cheeks, and forehead; known as facial chloasma

7. Genitourinary system
   a. Dilatation of ureters and renal pelvis due to progesterone and pressure from the enlarging uterus
   b. Increased glomerular filtration rate (GFR) and renal plasma flow (RPF) early in pregnancy; GFR is elevated until delivery, while RPF returns to a near-normal level by term
   c. Increased clearance of urea and creatinine due to increased renal function
   d. Decreased blood urea and nonprotein nitrogen values due to increased renal function

e. Glucosuria from increased glomerular filtration without an increase in tubular reabsorptive capacity
f. Decreased bladder tone
g. Sodium retention due to hormonal influences
h. Increased dimensions of uterus: from approximately 6.5 to 32 cm long; from 4 to 24 cm wide; from 2.5 to 22 cm in depth; from approximately 65 g to 1,200 g in weight; from approximately 1.5 ml to 5,000 ml in volume
i. Hypertrophy of uterine muscle cells by 5 to 10 times normal
j. Increased vascularity, edema, hypertrophy, and hyperplasia of the cervical glands
k. Increased vaginal secretions with a pH of 3.5 to 6
l. Cessation of ovulation and maturation of new follicles
m. Thickening of vaginal mucosa, loosening of vaginal connective tissue, and hypertrophy of small muscle cells

C. **Psychological adaptations to pregnancy: A woman's responses to pregnancy vary for many reasons, including hormonal changes, altered body image, and anticipated role changes. Cultural/sociologic background, emotional makeup, and reaction(s) to pregnancy are also factors. Common responses include:**
1. Ambivalence. Fear of pending role changes, unresolved emotional conflicts with one's own mother, fear of labor and delivery, and/or the need to alter career plans cause mixed feelings, even when pregnancy was planned.
2. Acceptance. As the pregnancy progresses, the woman's changing physical appearance, quickening, and hearing of fetal heart tones help her accept the pregnancy and perceive the fetus as real.
3. Introversion. The woman may turn her attention towards herself to prepare for the birth. This is normal; however, it may be interpreted by the partner as rejection, straining the relationship.
4. Emotional lability. Wide mood swings can strain marital or familial relationships. Subsequent feelings of inadequacy and confusion in spouse or family members may cause him/them to withdraw, thus adding to the woman's sense of rejection.

D. **Common discomforts of pregnancy, first trimester**
1. Nausea and vomiting; referred to as "morning sickness," but symptoms may occur at any time.
    a. Causes: hormonal changes, fatigue, emotional factors, and changes in carbohydrate metabolism
    b. Interventions: avoiding greasy, highly seasoned food; eating small, frequent meals; eating dry toast or crackers before rising in the morning
2. Nasal stuffiness/discharge and obstruction
    a. Cause: edema of the nasal mucosa caused by elevated estrogen levels
    b. Interventions: use of a cool-air vaporizer

    3.   Breast enlargement and tenderness
        a.   Cause: increased estrogen and progesterone levels
        b.   Interventions: wearing a well-fitted, support bra
    4.   Urinary frequency and urgency
        a.   Cause: pressure of the enlarging uterus on the bladder
        b.   When the uterus rises into the abdominal cavity around the 12th week, symptoms disappear; they recur in the third trimester as the uterus again presses on the bladder
        c.   Interventions: decreasing fluid intake in evening to reduce nocturia; limiting caffeine-containing fluids; responding to urge to void immediately to avoid bladder distention and urinary stasis; performing kegel exercises; promptly reporting any signs of urinary tract infection
    5.   Increased vaginal discharge (leukorrhea)
        a.   Cause: hyperplasia of vaginal mucosa and increased mucus production by the endocervical glands
        b.   Interventions: meticulous daily bathing and wearing absorbent cotton underwear

E. Common discomforts of pregnancy, second and third trimesters
    1.   Heartburn
        a.   Causes: relaxation of the cardiac sphincter, decreased gastrointestinal motility, increased production of progesterone, and gastric displacement
        b.   Interventions: eating small, frequent meals, avoiding fatty or fried foods, remaining upright after eating, and using antacids that do not contain sodium bicarbonate
    2.   Hemorrhoids
        a.   Causes: pressure on the pelvic veins by the enlarging uterus, which interferes with venous circulation
        b.   Interventions: avoiding constipation, prolonged standing, and constrictive clothing; use of topical ointments, warm soaks, and anesthetic agents
    3.   Constipation
        a.   Causes: oral iron supplements, displacement of the intestines by the fetus, and bowel sluggishness caused by increased progesterone and steroid metabolism
        b.   Interventions: daily exercise, increased fluid intake, regular patterns of elimination, and increased dietary bulk
    4.   Backache
        a.   Causes: postural adjustments of pregnancy; curvature of the lumbosacral vertebrae increases as the uterus enlarges
        b.   Interventions: use of proper body mechanics, good posture, avoiding high heels
    5.   Leg cramps
        a.   Causes: pressure from the enlarging uterus, poor circulation, fatigue, and an imbalance of the calcium/phosphorus ratio

   b. Interventions: altering calcium/phosphorus intake, frequent rest periods
       with legs raised, wearing warm clothing
   c. Intervention during a leg cramp: pointing the toes up towards the leg
       while pressing down on the knee
6. Shortness of breath
   a. Cause: pressure of the uterus on the diaphragm
   b. Interventions: good posture while standing, use of semi-Fowler's
       position at night
7. Ankle edema
   a. Causes: poor venous return from the lower extremities; aggravated by
       prolonged sitting or standing and warm weather
   b. Interventions: avoiding tight garments, elevating legs during rest
       periods, and dorsiflexion of feet if standing/sitting for prolonged periods

F. Gestational age assessment/estimated date of confinement
1. Naegele's Rule: determines the estimated date of confinement (EDC) by
    subtracting three months from LMP (LMP: first day of *l*ast *m*enstrual
    *p*eriod) and adding seven days; e.g., Oct. 5 − three months =
    July 5 + seven days = July 12
2. Fetal movement (quickening) usually felt first between 16 and 22 weeks of
    gestation
3. Fetal heart sounds detected from 10 to 12 weeks of gestation with an
    ultrasonic Doppler; 16 to 20 weeks with a fetoscope
4. Crown-to-rump measurements detectable by ultrasonography, which can be
    used to assess fetal age until the fetal head can be defined. Biparietal
    diameter measurements can be made by approx. 12 to 13 weeks of
    gestation
5. Fundal height difficult to interpret; measurement can be affected by
    maternal weight, polyhydramnios, multiple gestation, and fetal size
   a. McDonald's rule: method of determining the duration of a pregnancy in
       either lunar months or weeks.
   b. McDonald's method: Place tape measure at the symphysis pubic notch
       and measure up over the fundus. Height of fundus (cm) × 2/7 =
       duration of pregnancy in lunar months; height of fundus (cm) × 8/7 =
       duration of pregnancy in weeks

G. Prenatal monitoring of fetal status
1. Amniocentesis: insertion of a spinal needle into the uterus transabdominally
    to aspirate amniotic fluid for analysis
   a. Performed after the 14th week, when there is sufficient fluid and the
       uterus has moved into the abdominal cavity
   b. Must be preceded by ultrasound to locate fetus, placenta, and fluid

    c. Must be followed by at least 30 minutes of monitoring fetal heart and uterine activity via an external fetal monitor

    d. May be complicated by maternal hemorrhage, infection, premature labor, fetal hemorrhage, and amnionitis

2. Amniotic fluid assessment

    a. Prenatal diagnosis of genetic disorders such as chromosomal aberrations, sex-linked disorders, inborn errors of metabolism, and neural tube defects

    b. Diagnosis and continued evaluation of isoimmune disease (Rh sensitization and ABO incompatibility)

    c. Gestational age assessment via a lecithin/sphingomyelin ratio, presence of phosphatidylglycerol, creatinine levels, or the delta optical density of bilirubinoid pigments

3. Non-stress test (NST): non-invasive test in which fetal heart acceleration in response to fetal movement is the desired outcome

    a. Provides immediate results simply and inexpensively without contraindications or complications

    b. Benefits clients at risk for uteroplacental insufficiency and altered fetal movements

    c. Starts between 32 and 34 weeks of gestation

    d. Nonreactive NST may indicate fetal hypoxia, fetal sleep cycle, or the effects of drugs when nonreactive

    e. NST interpretation:

NST result	Interpretation	Actions
Reactive	Two or more fetal heart rate (FHR) accelerations of 15 beats/min. lasting 15 seconds or more within a 20-minute period	Repeat NST weekly
Nonreactive	Tracing without FHR accelerations or with accelerations less than 15 beats/min. or lasting less than 15 seconds throughout any fetal movement during the test period	Repeat in 24 hours or perform a stress test immediately
Unsatisfactory	Quality of FHR recording not adequate for interpretation	Repeat in 24 hours or perform a stress test immediately

4. Stress test (oxytocin challenge test, OCT): method of evaluating a fetus' ability to withstand the physiologic stress of an oxytocin-induced contraction

    a. Involves I.V. administration of oxytocin, usually starting at 0.5 mU/min. and increasing by 0.5 mU/min at 15- to 20-minute intervals until three high-quality uterine contractions are obtained within a 10-minute period

    b. Applies to clients at risk for placental insufficiency or fetal compromise from diabetes, heart disease, hypertension, history of previous stillbirth, renal disease, or a nonreactive NST

c. Does not apply to those with previous classical cesarean section, third-trimester bleeding, and clients at high risk for preterm labor
d. Starts at 32 to 34 weeks
e. Requires FHR pattern evaluation for early, late, and variable decelerations
f. Stress test interpretation:

OCT result	Interpretation	Action
Negative	No late decelerations; contraction frequency of three per 10 minutes Fetus would probably survive labor if it occurred within 1 week	No further action needed at this time
Positive	Persistent and consistent late decelerations occurring with more than half of contractions	Induce labor; fetus is at risk for perinatal morbidity and mortality
Suspicious	Late decelerations occurring with less than half of contractions after an adequate contraction pattern is established	Repeat test in 24 hours
Hyperstimulation	Late decelerations occurring with excessive uterine activity (more often than every 2 minutes, or more than 90 seconds long)	Repeat test in 24 hours
Unsatisfactory	Poor monitor tracing or uterine contraction pattern	Repeat test in 24 hours

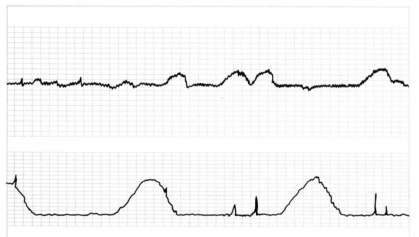

A fetal monitor strip is a recording of fetal heart rate (FHR) and maternal uterine contractions. The top strip shows a baseline FHR of 130 beats per minute with acceleration of at least 15 beats per minute lasting 15 minutes with each fetal movement. The bottom strip shows 3 uterine contractions in 8 minutes with no late decelerations of fetal heart rate. The strips are an example of a negative CST and reactive NST.

5. Nipple stimulation stress test (breast self-stimulation test)
   a. Stimulation of the nipples induces contractions by activating touch/sensory receptors in the areola, triggering the release of oxytocin by the posterior pituitary gland
   b. Breasts can be stimulated by nipple-rolling or applying warm washcloths to one nipple
   c. Test is noninvasive, less expensive, and less time-consuming than the OCT, but carries the risk of hyperstimulation, which is embarrassing to some clients
   d. Reactive pattern during test is the same as for reactive NST result
   e. Positive breast stimulation stress test results are the same as for positive OCT result
6. Daily fetal movement count
   a. The mother can identify approximately 90% of all fetal movements
   b. Fetal reactivity is affected by drugs, cigarettes, sound, time of day, sleep patterns, and blood glucose levels
   c. Researchers differ on the number of movements/hour that indicate positive fetal status. Generally, two or more movements/hour indicate fetal well-being.
7. Chorionic villi sampling: removal and analysis of a small tissue specimen from the fetal portion of the placenta to determine the genetic makeup of the fetus
   a. Can be performed as early as the 8th week of gestation
   b. Since results are received more quickly than from amniocentesis, provides an earlier diagnosis, an earlier and safer abortion if chosen, and less social and psychological stress
   c. Carries risk of spontaneous abortion, infection, hematoma, and intrauterine death
8. Ultrasonography
   a. Ultrasonic sound waves are reflected differently by tissues of different densities. Signals are amplified and displayed on an oscilloscope or screen.
   b. Test is noninvasive, painless, and provides immediate results without harm to fetus or mother
   c. Clinical use of ultrasonography includes detection of fetal death, malformation, malpresentations, placental abnormalities, multiple gestation, and hydramnios/oligohydramnios

H. Maternal prenatal physical examination
1. Breasts examination
   a. Inspection
   b. Palpation
2. Abdomen examination
   a. Inspection
   b. Auscultation

  c. Percussion
  d. Palpation
 3. External genitalia examination
  a. Inspection of pubic hair, skin, labia, clitoris, urethral orifice, perineum, and anus
  b. Palpation of the mons pubis, inguinal lymphatics, labia, Skene's and Bartholin's glands
 4. Speculum examination
  a. Inspection of the cervix
  b. Papanicolaou smear
  c. Inspection of vaginal mucosa
 5. Bimanual abdominovaginal palpation
  a. Cervix
  b. Uterus
  c. Cul-de-sac
  d. Adnexal area
 6. Rectovaginal palpation
  a. Uterus
  b. Adnexal area
  c. Cul-de-sac
 7. Smears for cytology
  a. Cervical
  b. Endocervical
  c. Vaginal

I. Maternal medical/obstetrical history

 1. Past medical history
  a. Childhood diseases
  b. Past surgical procedures
  c. Past medical problems (e.g., hypertension, renal or cardiac disease)
 2. Family medical history
  a. History of multiple births, congenital diseases or deformities
  b. Significant medical history
 3. Present medical status
  a. Prescription and OTC medications taken
  b. Alcohol/tobacco/illicit drug use
  c. Condition(s) that could influence pregnancy (X-rays, viral infections)
  d. Presence of disease conditions (e.g., diabetes, cardiac disease)
 4. Obstetrical history
  a. Number of pregnancies, abortions(s) (spontaneous and induced), living children
  b. History of previous pregnancies (antepartum, intrapartum, and postpartum)
  c. Perinatal status of previous neonate(s)

    5. Present pregnancy
       a. First day of LMP
       b. Abnormal symptoms (cramping, vaginal bleeding)
       c. Attitude toward pregnancy
    6. Gynecologic history
       a. History of infections (cervical, vaginal, sexually transmitted)
       b. Age of menarche; typical menstrual cycle
       c. Use of contraceptives
    7. Partner's history
       a. Age, presence of genetic or medical disorders
       b. Alcohol or drug use
    8. Personal information
       a. Age, religion, economic status, educational level
       b. History of emotional or psychiatric disorders
       c. Dietary practices

J. Routine maternal prenatal laboratory testing
    1. Rubella titer to assess immunity to rubella
    2. Complete blood count (CBC) to detect anemia and/or infection
    3. Blood type, Rh, and abnormal antibodies to identify fetus at risk for erythroblastosis fetalis or hyperbilirubinemia
    4. VDRL to detect untreated syphilis
    5. Serum glucose to detect gestational diabetes
    6. Urinalysis and urine culture to test for glucose, protein, blood, acetone, and asymptomatic bacteriuria

K. Counseling the prenatal client
    1. Childbirth and parenthood education
       a. Classes address the learning needs of the parents-to-be
       b. Subjects include nutrition, labor and delivery, breathing exercises, and anesthesia/analgesia
    2. Dental care
       a. Dental check-up early in pregnancy encouraged
       b. Nausea and vomiting, heartburn, and hyperemia of gums may lead to poor oral hygiene and caries
       c. The calcium and phosphorus required by the fetus should come from the maternal diet, not maternal teeth. There is no truth to the belief that a woman loses a tooth for every pregnancy due to the drain on calcium from her teeth.
    3. Immunizations
       a. Immunizations with attenuated live viruses should not be given during pregnancy, due to their teratogenic effect on the developing embryo; includes mumps and rubella vaccines
       b. Vaccinations with killed viruses may be given during pregnancy; includes influenza, tetanus, and diptheria vaccines
    4. Clothing
       a. Clothes should be nonconstrictive

    b. Low-heeled shoes help prevent backache and poor balance

    c. Maternity girdles are rarely needed by most women. However, individuals with pendulous abdomens may benefit from decreased curvature of the spine

5. Danger signs to report immediately
   a. Severe vomiting
   b. Frequent and severe headaches
   c. Epigastric pain
   d. Fluid discharge from vagina
   e. Altered or absent fetal movements after quickening
   f. Swelling of fingers or face
   g. Visual disturbances
   h. Signs of infections (vaginal or urinary)
   i. Unusual or severe abdominal pain
   j. Convulsions or muscular irritability

6. Substance abuse
   a. The potential for gross structural fetal defects is greatest in the first trimester, during organogenesis
   b. Smoking causes vasoconstriction and alters maternal and fetal heart rate, blood pressure, and cardiac output
   c. Smoking increases the incidence of low-birth-weight infants
   d. Effects of alcohol and drugs on the fetus/neonate are discussed in Section VIII-M-6 & 7

7. Medications: all pregnant women must be advised to consult a physician before taking *any* medication

8. Sexuality
   a. Sexual behavior (coital and noncoital) is generally unrestricted in complication-free pregnancies
   b. Sexual desires may decrease during the first trimester from discomforts and fatigue
   c. Sexual desires may increase in the second trimester due to relief from discomforts. Woman may have greater sexual satisfaction than before pregnancy, due to vascular congestion of the pelvis
   d. Sexual desires may decrease in the third trimester from increasing fatigue and abdominal size

9. Physical activity
   a. Prenatal exercises increase muscle strength in preparation for delivery and promote restoration of muscle tone after delivery
   b. Kegel exercises strengthen the pubococcygeus muscle and increase its elasticity
   c. Employed pregnant women should check their work site for potential hazards
   d. Excessive physical strain and medical or obstetric complications can deter employment during pregnancy
   e. Seat belts should be worn low, under the abdomen

10. Breast care
   a. Proper breast support promotes comfort, retains breast shape, and prevents back sprain
   b. Women who plan to breastfeed should begin stretching and rolling their nipples 2 months before delivery

L. Nutrition during pregnancy
   1. Calories
      a. Requirement during pregnancy exceeds prepregnancy needs by 300 calories/day (from 2,100 kcal/day to 2,400 kcal/day)
      b. Extra calories support tissue synthesis by fetus and mother and meet increased basal metabolic needs
      c. Increased caloric intake is required for optimal utilization of protein and tissue growth
   2. Protein
      a. Requirement during pregnancy exceeds normal needs by 30 g/day (from 46 g/day to 76 g/day)
      b. Increased protein intake is needed for expansion of blood volume, tissue growth, and provision of adequate amino acids for fetal development
   3. Vitamins
      a. Intake of all vitamins should be increased
      b. Increase is needed for tissue synthesis and energy production
      c. Folic acid is particularly important; it promotes fetal growth and prevents anemia. Intake should be increased from 400 mg/day to 800 mg/day
      d. Sources of folic acid include green, leafy vegetables; eggs; milk; and whole-grain breads
   4. Minerals
      a. All minerals, especially iron, need to be increased
      b. Average American diet does not provide enough iron to prevent iron-deficiency anemia. Recommended supplemental iron intake is 30 to 60 mg/day
      c. Sodium restriction is no longer advocated. Sodium maintains fluid and electrolyte balance, since sodium metabolism is altered during pregnancy

M. Complications of pregnancy
   1. Hyperemesis gravidarum
      a. Definition: pernicious vomiting during pregnancy
      b. Pathophysiology: is linked to trophoblastic activity, gonadotropin production, and psychological factors
      c. Clinical manifestations: weight loss, alkalosis, fluid and electrolyte imbalance, dehydration, oliguria, metabolic acidosis, and jaundice
      d. Management: restoration of fluid and electrolyte balance, control of vomiting, and maintenance of adequate nutrition and rest

2. Hydatidiform mole
   a. Definition: developmental anomaly of the placenta that converts the chorionic villi into a mass of clear vesicles; embryo is rarely present
   b. Pathophysiology: unknown
   c. Clinical manifestations: disproportionate enlargement of the uterus, excessive nausea and vomiting, intermittent or continuous bright-red or brownish vaginal bleeding by 12th week of gestation, symptoms of pregnancy-induced hypertension before the 20th week of gestation, no fetal heart tones, no fetal skeleton seen by ultrasound and human chorionic gonadotropin (hCG) levels much higher than the norm
   d. Management: induced abortion if a spontaneous one does not occur; hysterectomy may be performed since the cancer rate is 15% in women of high parity and 35% in women over age 40; careful monitoring of hCG levels for 1 year; emotional support for couple grieving for lost pregnancy and unsure obstetrical and medical future
3. Placenta previa
   a. Definition: implantation of the placenta low in the uterus, occurring either in the lower uterine segment (low implantation), or occluding a portion of the cervical os (partial placenta previa), or totally occluding the cervical os (total placenta previa)

Placenta previa

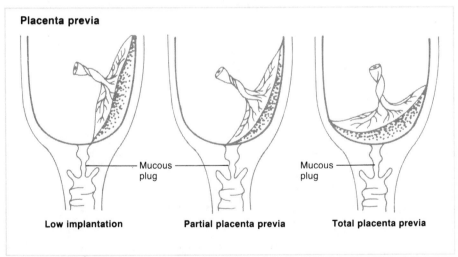

Low implantation   Partial placenta previa   Total placenta previa

   b. Pathophysiology: associated with uterine fibroid tumors and uterine scars from surgery. Placental villi are torn from the uterine wall as the lower uterine segment contracts and dilates in the third trimester. Uterine sinuses are exposed at the placental site and bleeding occurs
   c. Clinical manifestations: painless, bright-red vaginal bleeding, especially during the third trimester. Initial bleeding is scant, but may increase with each successive incident

    d. Management: depends upon when during gestation the first episode occurred and the amount of bleeding; management includes limiting maternal activities, monitoring all relevant vital signs, and providing emotional support

    e. Note: rectal or vaginal exams should not be performed unless a double set-up is available for delivery. Placenta can be located via ultrasound.

4. Abruptio placenta

    a. Definition: premature separation of the placenta from the uterine wall after the 20th to 24th week of pregnancy

Abruptio placenta

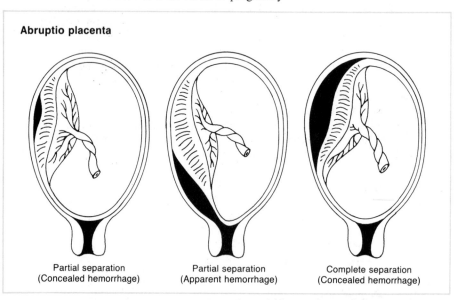

Partial separation
(Concealed hemorrhage)

Partial separation
(Apparent hemorrhage)

Complete separation
(Concealed hemorrhage)

Grade	Criteria
0	Occurrence of premature separation not apparent until placenta is examined after delivery. Maternal and fetal signs did not indicate presence of any difficulty.
1	Minimal separation, which causes vaginal bleeding and alterations in maternal vital signs. Symptoms of hemorrhagic shock or fetal distress do not appear.
2	Moderate degree of separation with signs of fetal distress. The uterus will be tense and painful when palpated.
3	Extreme separation, causing maternal shock and fetal death without immediate intervention.

    b. Pathophysiology: contributing factors include multiple pregnancy, hydramnios, decreased blood flow to the placenta, and trauma to the abdomen. Women with low serum folic acid levels, vascular or renal disease, and/or pregnancy-induced hypertension (PIH) are at risk.

    c. Clinical manifestations: hemorrhage, either concealed or apparent; shock; acute abdominal pain; rigid abdomen; uteroplacental insufficiency

    d. Management: monitor maternal vital signs, fetal heart rate, uterine contractions, vaginal bleeding, maternal lab values, fluid and electrolyte balance; provide emotional support. Likelihood of vaginal delivery depends on the degree of separation and timing of separation in labor. A cesarean delivery is indicated in moderate to severe placental separation. To determine the fetal and maternal outcome, the degrees of placental separation can be graded from 0 to 3

    e. Fetal implications: perinatal mortality depends on the degree of placental separation and fetal level of maturity; the most serious complications stem from hypoxia, prematurity, and anemia

    f. Maternal implications: mortality rate is approximately 6% and depends on the bleeding's severity, the presence of coagulation defects, hypofibrinogenemia, and the time lapse between placental separation and delivery. Postpartum clients are at risk for vascular spasm, intravascular clotting and/or hemorrhage, and renal failure from shock.

5. Polyhydramnios (hydramnios)

    a. Definition: presence of greater than 2,000 ml of amniotic fluid in the uterus; the fluid may have increased gradually (chronic type) or rapidly (acute type)

    b. Pathophysiology: exact cause unknown in approximately 35% of all cases. Associated with diabetes mellitus in approximately 25% of cases, and with erythroblastosis (10%), multiple gestation (10%), and congenital anomalies (20%)

    c. Clinical manifestations: depends on the length of gestation, the amount of amniotic fluid, and whether the disorder is chronic or acute. Symptoms include abdominal discomfort and slight dyspnea in mild cases; severe dyspnea, orthopnea, and edema of the vulva, legs, and abdomen in severe cases. In both cases, the uterus will be larger than expected for number of weeks of gestation, the fetal parts will be difficult to outline, and the fetal heart may be difficult to hear.

    d. Management: a high-protein, low-sodium diet, mild sedation, amniocentesis to remove excessive fluid, induction of labor if fetus is mature and symptoms are severe

    e. Fetal/neonatal implications: prolapsed cord at the rupture of membranes; increased incidence of malpresentations; increased perinatal mortality from fetal malformations and premature deliveries

    f. Maternal implications: shortness of breath, especially when the fluid exceeds 3,000 ml; edema of legs from compression of the vena cava; and increased incidence of postpartum hemorrhage

6. Oligohydramnios

    a. Definition: severely reduced and highly concentrated amniotic fluid

    b. Pathophysiology: associated with postmature infants, intrauterine growth retardation, and renal agenesis or obstruction in the fetal urinary tract

   c. Clinical manifestations: diagnosis made via ultrasonography
   d. Management: close medical supervision and prenatal monitoring of fetal status
   e. Fetal/neonatal implications: associated with renal anomalies, wrinkled, leathery skin, pulmonary hypoplasia, increased skeletal deformities, and fetal hypoxia
   f. Maternal implications: prolonged, dysfunctional labor usually beginning before term

7. Ectopic pregnancy
   a. Definition: implantation of the fertilized ovum outside the uterine cavity. Most ectopic pregnancies occur in a fallopian tube; other sites include the cervix, ovary, or abdominal cavity
   b. Pathophysiology: any condition that prevents or retards the passage of a fertilized ovum through the fallopian tube, such as hormonal factors, tubal damage from previous pelvic or tubal surgery, damage from pelvic inflammatory disease, tubal atony, tubal spasms, and malformed fallopian tubes
   c. Clinical manifestations: symptoms of early pregnancy, irregular vaginal bleeding, and dull abdominal pain on the affected side early in the pregnancy. As the pregnancy progresses, the tubes rupture, causing sudden and severe abdominal pain, syncope, and referred shoulder pain as the abdomen fills with blood; nausea and vomiting; shock if hemorrhage is profuse; hCG titers lower than normal
   d. Management: laparotomy to remove the affected tube or to perform a salpingostomy (incision into the tube to remove the pregnancy); emotional support for parents grieving over loss of pregnancy

8. Rh sensitization
   a. Definition: an antigen-antibody immunologic reaction within the body that occurs when an Rh-negative mother carries an Rh-positive fetus
   b. Pathophysiology: fetal red blood cells enter the maternal circulation and stimulate the production of Rh antibodies. In subsequent pregnancies, antibodies cross the placenta and enter the fetal circulation, causing erythroblastosis if the fetus is Rh positive.
   c. Clinical manifestations: increased concentration (optical density) of bilirubin and red blood cell breakdown products in the amniotic fluid
   d. Management: monitoring of the indirect Coombs' test, which measures the amount of antibodies in the maternal blood; delta optical density analysis of the amniotic fluid at 26 weeks, intrauterine transfusion, emotional support to parents, and possible early delivery of the fetus

9. Cystitis
   a. Definition: inflammation of the lower urinary tract
   b. Pathophysiology: caused by vesicoureteral reflux, urinary stasis, and compression of the ureters
   c. Clinical manifestations: burning upon urination; urinary urgency and frequency, and temperature of 101°F. (38.4°C.)

  d. Management: good hygiene, increased fluid intake, urine culture to
      identify organism. Oral sulfonamides may be used in early pregnancy;
      use in later pregnancy can cause neonatal hyperbilirubinemia and
      kernicterus. Ampicillin and Furadantin are appropriate in later
      pregnancy.
10. Pyelonephritis
  a. Definition: inflammation of the upper urinary tract
  b. Pathophysiology: ureteritis, edema of the renal parenchyma, and
      ureteral swelling
  c. Clinical manifestations: severe colicky pain, vomiting, dehydration,
      sudden onset with chills, temperature 103° to 105°F. (39.6° to 40.6°C.),
      flank pain
  d. Management: urine culture, hospitalization, I.V. antibiotics, monitoring
      of intake and output, vital signs, laboratory reports, fetal status
11. Monilial infections
  a. Definition: vaginal yeast infection
  b. Causative organism: *Candida albicans*
  c. Clinical manifestations: thick, white, pruritic vaginal discharge
      accompanied by dysuria and dyspareunia
  d. Management: drug therapy (Mycostatin, clotrimazole), review of
      personal hygiene, abstinence from intercourse or use of condom until
      infection is cured
  e. Fetal/neonatal implications: if infection is not cured before delivery, the
      fetus may contract thrush by direct contact with the organism in the
      vagina
  f. Clients at risk: women with poorly controlled diabetes mellitus or those
      on steroid or antibiotic therapy
12. Miscarriage
  a. Definition: spontaneous termination of a pregnancy before the 20th
      week of gestation; a spontaneous abortion
  b. Pathophysiology: greater than 50% are caused by abnormalities in
      fetoplacental development; the remainder are from maternal or unknown
      causes
  c. Clinical manifestations: severity of symptoms depends on the
      gestational age at the time of miscarriage; symptoms include uterine
      cramping, vaginal bleeding, weakly positive urine pregnancy test,
      minimal or absent estrogen, hCH, and progesterone titers
  d. Management: varies with type and stage of spontaneous abortion

Type/stage	Management
Threatened miscarriage	Limit activities for 24 to 48 hours. Coitus restricted approximately 2 weeks
Imminent and incomplete	Dilatation and curettage to ensure emptying of uterus
Complete	If uterus emptied on its own and there are no signs of infection, no further intervention is needed.

13. Pregnancy-induced hypertension (PIH)
    a. Definition: disorder of pregnancy characterized by hypertension, proteinuria, and edema. PIH was once called preeclampsia (before convulsions) and eclampsia (with convulsions)
    b. Pathophysiology: predisposing factors include diabetes mellitus, malnutrition, hydramnios, hypertension, renal disease, obesity, multiple pregnancy, hydatidiform mole, and familial tendency
    c. Clinical manifestations: hypertension is defined as blood pressure over 140/90, a systolic increase of 30 mm Hg over prepregnancy levels, or a diastolic increase of 15 mm Hg over prepregnancy levels. Proteinuria is measured as 0.5 g/liter/24 hours, or +1 or +2 via dipstick. Increased generalized edema is connected with a sudden weight gain of greater than 2 lbs/week. PIH usually appears between the 20th and 24th week of gestation and disappears by 42 days postdelivery. A final diagnosis is usually deferred until blood pressure returns to normal after delivery; if blood pressure remains elevated, chronic hypertension, either alone or superimposed upon PIH, may be the cause.
    d. Additional manifestations: increased BUN, creatinine, and uric acid levels; frontal headaches, blurred vision, hyperreflexia, nausea, vomiting, irritability, cerebral disturbances, and epigastric pain
    e. Maternal implications: disorder may progress to convulsions (eclampsia); maternal mortality rate in eclampsia is approximately 10 to 15%, usually resulting from intracranial hemorrhage and congestive heart failure
    f. Severe complications of eclampsia: cerebral edema, maternal cerebrovascular accident, abruptio placenta with or without disseminated intravascular coagulation (DIC), and fetal death
    g. Management: high-protein diet, with avoidance of excessively salty foods; bed rest in a left lateral position; monitoring of blood pressure, fetal heart rate, edema, proteinuria, and signs of pending eclampsia; administration of magnesium sulfate, a neuromuscular sedative that decreases the amount of acetylcholine produced by motor nerves, thus preventing seizures. Early signs of toxicity include decreased reflexes (especially patellar reflex), muscle flaccidity, central nervous system depression, and decreased renal functions. The antidote for magnesium sulfate is calcium gluconate or calcium chloride. Urine output must be 30 ml/hour, because 99% of the drug is excreted by the kidney.

N. High-risk pregnancy
1. Maternal age: a pregnant women is classified as high risk if she is:
   a. age 16 or younger
   b. a nullipara age 35 or older
   c. a multipara age 40 or older

2. Parity factors: a pregnant woman is classified as high risk if her parity fits one of these categories:
   a. Eight years or more since last pregnancy
   b. High parity (five or more)
   c. Pregnancy occurs within 3 months of last delivery
3. Diabetes
   a. A disorder of fat, carbohydrate, and protein metabolism caused by a relative or complete lack of insulin secretion by the beta cells of the pancreas. Insulin-dependent diabetes mellitus (IDDM) predates the pregnancy, gestational diabetes mellitus (form of non-insulin dependent diabetes mellitus [NIDDM]) may begin at pregnancy
   b. Pathophysiology: gestational diabetes mellitus (IDDM) occurs when the woman's pancreas, stressed by the normal adaptations to pregnancy, cannot meet the increased demands for insulin
   c. Clinical manifestations: glucosuria and thirst first appearing around the 18th to 20th week of gestation
   d. Management of gestational diabetes: careful monitoring of blood glucose levels; diet; exercise and insulin administration. Oral hypoglycemic agents are contraindicated in pregnancy due to their adverse effects on the fetus and newborn. Women with insulin-dependent diabetes mellitus are more prone to wide fluctuations in blood glucose levels
   e. Maternal implications: women with gestational diabetes have a 30 to 40% chance of developing diabetes mellitus within 1 to 25 years
   f. Fetal/neonatal implications: mild insulin-dependent diabetes can cause hydramnios, macrosomia, PIH, and fetal death. Advanced insulin-dependent diabetes can cause spontaneous abortion, intrauterine fetal death, and neonatal death
   g. Note: the two most important factors related to pregnancy outcome are the age of onset and duration of diabetes mellitus, not the daily insulin requirements
4. Sickle cell anemia
   a. Definition: a recessive autosomal disorder in which red blood cells become sickle-shaped
   b. Pathophysiology: causes vascular obstruction in the capillaries, which leads to anemia
   c. Maternal implications: increased incidence of PIH, urinary tract infections, congestive heart failure, pneumonia, pulmonary infarction, crisis, and postpartum hemorrhage
   d. Fetal/neonate implications: neonates of women with sickle cell anemia are at risk for intrauterine growth retardation and perinatal fetal death from spontaneous abortion and prematurity
   e. Management: monitoring of hemoglobin and hematocrit levels; avoidance of contributing factors, such as dehydration, stress, hypoxia, infection, acidosis, and sudden cooling; monitoring for thrombophlebitis (positive Homans' sign); folic acid supplementation to decrease

erythropoietic demands and capillary stasis. Heparin may be administered. Coumadin is contraindicated because it can cross the placenta and harm the fetus

5. Cardiac disease
   a. Definition: impaired cardiac function, primarily from congenital or rheumatic heart disease. Congenital: atrial septal defect, ventricular septal defect, pulmonary stenosis, coarctation of aorta. Rheumatic: endocarditis with scar tissue formation on mitral, aortic, or tricuspid valve(s) with resulting stenosis and/or regurgitation
   b. Pathophysiology: depends on location and severity of defect. For example, valvular stenosis decreases blood flow through valve, increasing workload on heart chambers located before stenotic valve. Regurgitation permits blood to leak through incompletely closed valve, increasing workload on heart chambers on either side of affected valve
   c. Clinical manifestations: dyspnea, tachycardia, diastolic murmur at the heart apex, cough, hemoptysis, and rales at the lung bases
   d. Maternal implications: pregnancy taxes a woman's cardiopulmonary system (Refer to Section IV-B-1). The normal heart can compensate for increased demands, but if myocardial or valvular disease develops, or if the mother has a congenital heart defect, cardiac decomposition may occur. Women with cardiac disorders are at greatest risk when blood volume peaks between the 28th and 32nd week of gestation
   e. Fetal neonatal implications: decreased placental perfusion leading to intrauterine growth retardation, fetal distress, prematurity
   f. Management: close medical supervision, limitation of activities, adequate rest, limited sodium intake, and antibiotics as prophylactic measures
   g. Note: a successful pregnancy depends on the type and extent of the disease. Heart disease in pregnancy can be divided into four categories, as shown below. Women in class I or II can expect a successful pregnancy and delivery. Women in class III must maintain almost complete bed rest to complete the pregnancy. Women in class IV are poor candidates for pregnancy.

Class	Description
I	Patients have unrestricted physical activity. Ordinary activity causes no discomfort. There are no symptoms of cardiac insufficiency or anginal pain.
II	Patients have a slight limitation of physical activity. Ordinary activity causes excessive fatigue, palpitations, dyspnea, or anginal pain.
III	Patients have a moderate to marked limitation of activity. With less than ordinary activity, they experience excessive fatigue, palpitation, dyspnea, or anginal pain.
IV	Patients cannot engage in any physical activity without discomfort. Symptoms of cardiac insufficiency or anginal pain occur even at rest.

6. Poor obstetrical history: a woman defined as having a poor obstetrical history may fall into one of the following high-risk categories:
   a. Two or more previous premature deliveries
   b. Two or more consecutive miscarriages
   c. One or more stillbirths at term
   d. One or more gross anomalies
   e. Previous birth defects
   f. History of Dystocia
   g. Poor self-care practices
7. Drug-addicted mother
   a. The number of pregnant drug abusers has increased during the last decade
   b. Drug addiction may be compounded by malnutrition, alcoholism, sexually transmitted diseases, and/or poor self-image
   c. Maternal complications include cellulitis, septic phlebitis, superficial abscesses, and acute pulmonary edema
   d. Three out of four pregnant addicts do not seek prenatal care
   e. Clients should receive long-term counseling and rehabilitation (social, medical, psychiatric, and vocational)
   f. Fetal/neonatal implications are discussed in Section VIII-M-7

Points to Remember

Comprehensive prenatal care is essential for the health of the expectant woman and her unborn child.

Obtaining a thorough maternal physical examination and history increases the chances of a successful pregnancy.

Pregnancy represents a developmental crisis for the woman and her family.

The nurse must understand the normal physical and psychological changes of pregnancy to identify deviations from the norm.

Glossary

Adnexal area—accessory parts of the uterus, ovaries, and fallopian tubes

Cul-de-sac—a pouch formed by a fold of the peritoneum between the anterior wall of the rectum and the posterior wall of the uterus; also known as Douglas' cul-de-sac

Homans' sign—early sign of thrombophlebitis; calf pain occurs when the leg is extended and the foot dorsiflexed

Lecithin/sphingomyelin—phospholipids that reduce surface tension and increase pulmonary tissue elasticity; phospholipids are also referred to as surfactants.

Leukorrhea—whitish or yellowish vaginal discharge

Labor and Delivery

Learning Objectives

After studying this section, the reader should be able to:

● Differentiate between the four stages of labor.

● Describe the nurse's role when caring for a client in labor.

● Describe a woman's physiologic and psychological responses to labor.

● Describe methods of assessing fetal status during labor.

● List possible complications during labor and delivery.

V. Labor and Delivery

A. Initiation of labor. Theories regarding labor initiation include:

1. Oxytocin stimulation: although it has not been proven that either maternal or fetal oxytocin initiates labor, the myometrium of a woman at term is increasingly sensitive to oxytocin, possibly due to the stimulating effects of estrogen
2. Progesterone withdrawal: decreased progesterone metabolism in the fetus (and possibly in the mother) may stimulate prostaglandin synthesis in the chorioamnion, resulting in increased uterine contractility
3. Estrogen stimulation: estrogen irritates the myometrium; promotes prostaglandin synthesis, which increases myometrial muscle contraction; and helps transmit impulses over the uterine muscle after the muscle cells are irritated and the muscle contracts
4. Fetal cortisol: cortisol may alter the biochemistry of the fetal membrane
5. Distention: as the uterus stretches, the production, release, and myometrial concentrations of prostaglandin F increase
6. Fetal membrane phospholipid-arachidonic acid-prostaglandin: prostaglandin, which is present in blood and amniotic fluid, stimulates the smooth muscle of the myometrium to contract

B. Premonitory signs of labor

1. Lightening: the descent of the fetus into the pelvis; usually occurs 2 to 3 weeks before term in primigravidas and later or during labor in the multipara
2. Braxton-Hicks contractions: irregular and intermittent contractions that occur throughout pregnancy; they become uncomfortable and produce "false labor"
3. Cervical changes: several days before initiation of labor, the cervix softens, begins to efface, and dilates slightly
4. Bloody show: expulsion of mucous plug from the cervix, resulting in pink-tinged secretions
5. Rupture of membranes (ROM): occurs before onset of labor in approximately 12% of women. Labor begins within 24 hours for about 80% of these women
6. Burst of energy: some women experience a sudden burst of energy prior to the onset of labor; often manifested by housecleaning activities and called the "nesting instinct"

C. Differentiation between true and false labor

True labor	False labor
• Regular contractions	• Irregular contractions
• Discomfort begins in the back and spreads to the abdomen	• Discomfort localized in abdomen
• Progressive cervical dilatation and effacement	• No change
• Intervals between contractions gradually shorten	• No change or irregular change
• Intensity of contractions increases with ambulation	• Ambulating has no effect on contractions
• Contractions increase in duration and intensity	• Usually no change

D. Stages of labor: first stage
1. The first stage is measured from the onset of true labor to complete dilatation of the cervix
2. Length ranges from 6 to 18 hours in a primigravida, 2 to 10 hours in a multipara. It is divided into three phases: latent, active, and transitional
3. Latent phase
   a. Dilatation measures from zero to 3 cm; contractions are irregular
   b. Mother may feel anticipation, excitement, and/or apprehension about pending delivery
4. Active phase
   a. Dilatation measures from 4 to 7 cm; contractions are approximately 5 to 8 minutes apart, lasting 45 to 60 seconds and moderate to strong in intensity
   b. Mother becomes serious and concerned about the progress of labor; she may ask for pain medication or use breathing techniques
5. Transitional phase
   a. Dilatation measures from 8 to 10 cm; contractions are approximately 1 to 2 minutes apart, lasting 60 to 90 seconds and strong in intensity
   b. Mother may lose control, thrash in bed, groan, or cry out

E. Stages of labor: second stage
1. The second stage extends from the time of complete dilatation to delivery of the infant
2. Length ranges from 2 to 60 minutes, with an average of 20 contractions for the primigravida and 20 minutes or 10 contractions for the multigravida
3. Maternal behavior changes from coping with contractions to actively pushing; mother may become exhausted

F. Stages of labor: third stage
1. The third stage extends from the delivery of the infant to the expulsion of the placenta
2. Length ranges from approximately 5 to 30 minutes
3. Mother may focus on condition of infant; may experience discomfort due to uterine contractions before expulsion of placenta

G. Stages of labor: fourth stage
1. The fourth stage is the first hour postdelivery
2. Primary activity is promotion of maternal-infant bonding

H. Nursing interventions during labor and delivery
1. Provide emotional support to mother and coach
2. Inform mother of labor progress regarding dilatation, station, effacement, and fetal well-being
3. Monitor frequency, duration, and strength of contractions
4. Monitor fetal heart rate during and between contractions, noting rate, accelerations, decelerations, and variability
5. Monitor and record I.V. fluid intake
6. Assess need for pain medication and evaluate effectiveness of medication administered
7. Monitor maternal vital signs frequently
8. Maintain aseptic technique
9. Maintain client's comfort via mouth care, ice chips, change of bed linen
10. Assist with breathing techniques
11. Encourage rest between contractions
12. Explain all nursing activities and equipment before initiation of action
13. Observe for rupture of membranes (ROM), noting color, odor, amount, and consistency of amniotic fluid
14. Observe for prolapsed cord and check fetal heart immediately after ROM
15. Observe perineum for show and bulging
16. Monitor urine output
17. Assess for signs of hypotensive supine syndrome; if blood pressure falls:
    a. Position client on left side
    b. Increase primary I.V. flow rate
    c. Administer oxygen via face mask at 6 to 10 liters/min

I. Mechanisms of labor
1. Engagement: the fetal head is considered "engaged" when the biparietal diameter passes the pelvic inlet
2. Descent: movement of the presenting part through the pelvis
3. Flexion: flexing of the head so that the fetal chin moves closer to the chest
4. Internal rotation: rotation of the head to pass through the ischial spines
5. Extension: extension of the fetal head as it passes under the symphysis pubis
6. External rotation: the head is externally rotated as the shoulders rotate to the anteroposterior position in the pelvis

J. Factors affecting the labor process: passenger
1. Fetal head: size and presence of molding

Head at term showing diameters

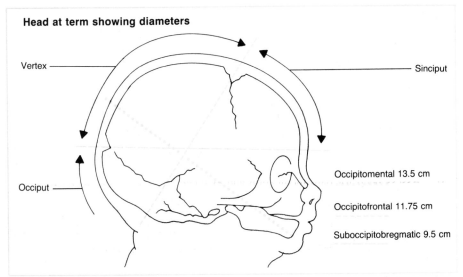

Vertex

Sinciput

Occiput

Occipitomental 13.5 cm

Occipitofrontal 11.75 cm

Suboccipitobregmatic 9.5 cm

2. Fetal lie: relationship of the long axis (spine) of the fetus to the long axis of the mother
   a. Longitudinal lie: the long axis of the fetus is parallel to the long axis of the mother
   b. Transverse lie: the long axis of the fetus is perpendicular to the long axis of the mother
3. Fetal presentation: portion of the fetus that enters the pelvic passageway first
   a. Cephalic: vertex, face, and brow
   b. Breech: frank, single or double-footling, and complete
   c. Shoulder: transverse lie that must be turned before delivery

Molding of Head: Cephalic Presentations

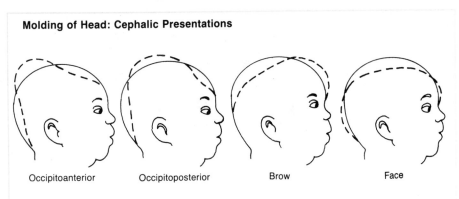

Occipitoanterior   Occipitoposterior   Brow   Face

(Note: soft tissues of face become edematous and ecchymotic in face presentations).

Fetal position

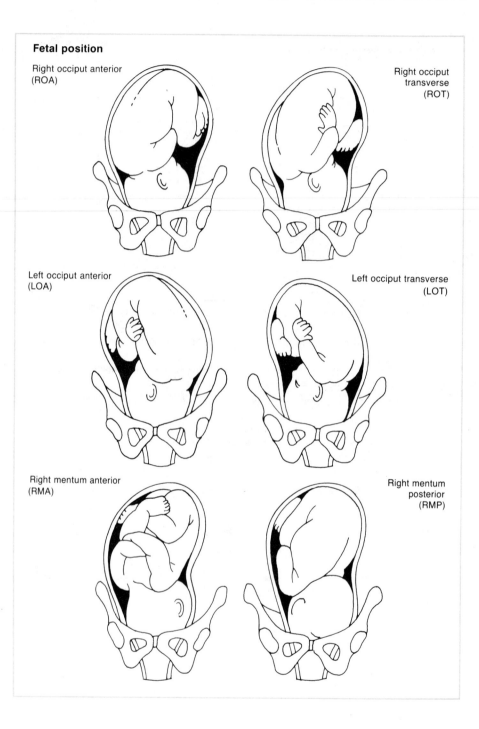

Right occiput anterior
(ROA)

Right occiput
transverse
(ROT)

Left occiput anterior
(LOA)

Left occiput transverse
(LOT)

Right mentum anterior
(RMA)

Right mentum
posterior
(RMP)

Fetal position continued

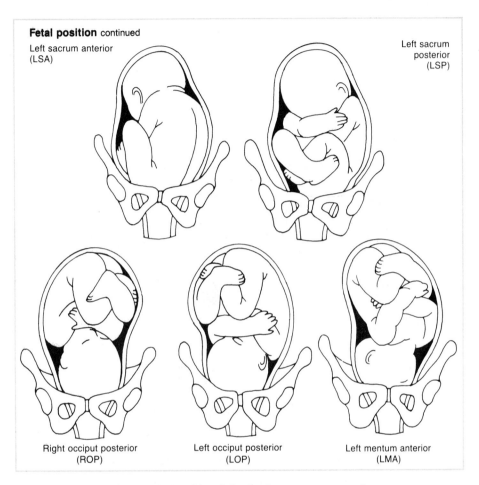

Left sacrum anterior (LSA)

Left sacrum posterior (LSP)

Right occiput posterior (ROP)

Left occiput posterior (LOP)

Left mentum anterior (LMA)

4. Fetal attitude: relationship of the fetal parts to one another
5. Fetal position: relationship of landmark on the presenting part to the front, back, and sides of the maternal pelvis. Notations used to designate fetal positions:
   a. Side of maternal pelvis: right (R) or left (L)
   b. Landmark on the presenting part: occiput (O), mentum (M), sacrum (S), acromion process (A)
   c. Position of the landmark on the pelvis: anterior (A), posterior (P), transverse (T)
   d. Positions in vertex presentations: ROA,ROT,ROP,LOA,LOT,LOP
   e. Positions in face presentation: RMA,RMT,RMP,LMA,LMT,LMP
   f. Positions in breech presentation: RSA,RST,RSP,LSA,LST,LSP

Leopold's maneuvers

First maneuver
Palpation of superior pole.

Second maneuver
Palpation of fetal back and small parts.

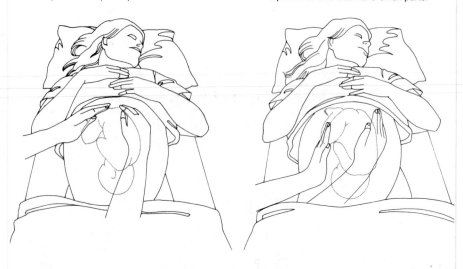

Third maneuver
Assessment of presenting part: cephalic prominence, flexion, and engagement.

Fourth maneuver
Palpation of cephalic prominence to determine descent and flexion.

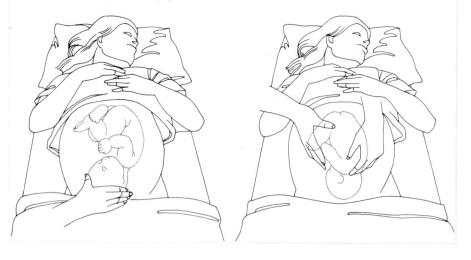

6. Leopold's maneuvers: a four-step process of abdominal palpation to determine fetal position and presentation
   a. First maneuver: palpation of the fundus to identify occupying fetal part. The fetal head is firm, rounded, and freely movable; the breech is softer, less regular, and moves with the trunk.
   b. Second maneuver: abdominal palpation to identify the location of the fetal back. The back feels firm, smooth, and convex, while the front of the fetus is soft, irregular, and concave.
   c. Third maneuver: grasping of the lower portion of the abdomen above the symphysis pubis to identify the fetal part presenting over the inlet. An unengaged fetal head can be rocked from side to side. This maneuver helps determine the attitude of the unengaged fetal head.
   d. Fourth maneuver: movement of fingers down both sides of the uterus to assess the descent of the presenting part into the pelvis. As the fingers move downward, greater resistance will be met on the cephalic prominence (brow) side. This maneuver helps determine whether the fetal head is flexed.

K. Factors affecting the labor process: passageway
  1. Type of pelvis: names derived from structure of inlet
     a. Gynecoid: rounded inlet; 50% of female pelves
     b. Android: heart-shaped inlet; normal male pelvis; 20% of female pelves
     c. Anthropoid: oval inlet; 25% of female pelves
     d. Platypelloid: transverse oval inlet; 5% of female pelves
  2. Structure of the pelvis: pelvic joints
     a. Symphysis pubis
     b. Right sacroiliac joint
     c. Left sacroiliac joint
     d. Sacrococcygeal joint
  3. Structure of the pelvis: pelvic bones
     a. Ilium
     b. Ischium
     c. Sacrum
     d. Coccyx
  4. Structure of the pelvis: true vs. false pelvis
     a. False pelvis is that portion above the pelvic inlet
     b. True pelvis is composed of the pelvic inlet, pelvic cavity, and pelvic outlet
  5. Pelvic diameters: inlet
     a. Anteroposterior diameters: true conjugate, 11 cm or greater; diagonal conjugate, 12.5 to 13 cm; obstetric conjugate, 12.5 to 13 cm
     b. Transverse diameter: 13.5 cm or greater
     c. Oblique diameter: 12.75 cm or greater

6. Pelvic diameters: outlet
   a. Anteroposterior diameter: approximately 11.9 cm
   b. Transverse or intertuberous diameter: 10 to 11 cm
   c. Posterior sagittal diameter: approximately 9 cm
7. Soft tissues
   a. Lower uterine segment: segment of uterus that expands to accommodate intrauterine contents as the walls of the upper segment thicken
   b. Cervix: the cervix is drawn upward and over the presenting part as it descends
   c. Vaginal canal: the vagina distends to accommodate passage of the fetus

L. Factors affecting the labor process: powers
1. Uterine contractions: the primary power; it causes complete effacement and dilatation of the cervix
2. Voluntary bearing down: use of abdominal muscles to push during the second stage of labor

M. Factors affecting the labor process: placental positioning (Refer to Section IV-M-3)

N. Factors affecting the labor process: psychological response. Factors that may influence a woman's psychological response to the emotional and physical crisis of labor include:
1. Support systems
2. Preparation for childbirth
3. Past experiences
4. Coping mechanisms
5. Accomplishment of the tasks of pregnancy

O. Maternal physiologic responses to labor
1. Cardiovascular system
   a. Increased intrathoracic pressure during pushing in the second stage
   b. Increased peripheral resistance during contractions, leading to increased blood pressure and decreased pulse
   c. Increased cardiac output
2. Fluid and electrolyte balance
   a. Insensible water loss from diaphoresis and hyperventilation
   b. Increased evaporative water volume from increased respiratory rate
3. Respiratory system
   a. Increased oxygen consumption
   b. Increased respiratory rate
4. Hemopoietic system
   a. Increased plasma fibrinogen and leukocytes
   b. Decreased blood coagulation time and blood glucose levels

5. Gastrointestinal system
   a. Decreased gastric motility and absorption
   b. Prolonged gastric emptying time
6. Renal system
   a. Displacement of base of bladder forward and upward at engagement
   b. Possible proteinuria due to muscle breakdown
   c. Possible impaired drainage of blood and lymph from the base of the
      bladder due to edema caused by the presenting part

P. Maternal evaluation during labor
1. Manifestations of progress: the client should be monitored for
   a. Dilatation: the opening of the external os from closed to 10 cm dilated
   b. Effacement: the thinning and shortening of the cervix, measured from
      0 (thick) to 100% effaced (paper thin)
   c. Station: relationship of the presenting part to the pelvic ischial spines.
      When the presenting part is even with the ischial spines, it is at 0
      station; above the ischial spines, it is -3, -2, -1; below the ischial
      spines, it is $+1$, $+2$, $+3$.

Measuring Fetal Station

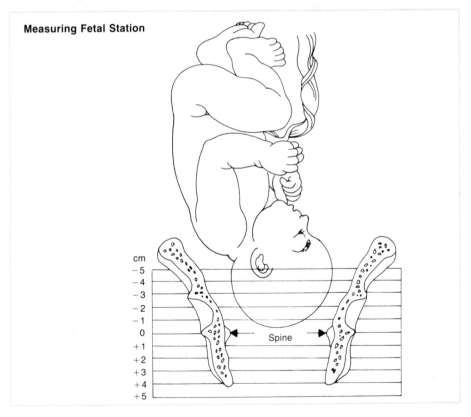

2.   Elimination: the client should void every 2 hours; a full bladder can impede fetal descent and cause dysfunctional labor
3.   Hydration: the client should be monitored for signs of dehydration, such as poor skin turgor, decreased urine output, and dry mucous membranes
4.   Contractions: the client can be monitored for presence of tetanic contractions (sustained, prolonged contractions with little rest between) by external pressure transducer

Q. Fetal evaluation during labor: external electronic monitoring
1.   Fetal heart rate (FHR) can be noninvasively monitored either intermittently with a hand-held device or continuously with a large fetal monitor
2.   The intensity and frequency of the contractions can be monitored continuously by use of a tocodynamometer (toco), a pressure device that, in response to uterine contractions, transfers an electrical impulse to the monitor and creates a readout.
3.   Advantages of external electronic monitoring:
     a.   Evaluates decreased variability and periodic changes
     b.   Grossly evaluates contractions
     c.   Provides a permanent record
4.   Disadvantages of external electronic monitoring
     a.   Readout is subject to artifacts
     b.   Fetal heart rate monitor and toco can be uncomfortable for the client
     c.   External monitor cannot assess variability unless decreased

R. Fetal evaluation during labor: internal electronic monitoring
1.   Internal spiral electrode: small electrode applied to the epidermis of the presenting part.
     a.   Provides a continuous recording of FHR
     b.   Demonstrates true baseline variability, periodic changes, and accurate baseline
2.   Intrauterine pressure catheter
     a.   Inserted into the uterine cavity near the fetal small parts
     b.   Provides a continuous, sensitive recording of the intensity and frequency of contractions
3.   Advantages of internal electronic monitoring
     a.   Provides the most precise assessment of FHR and uterine contractions
     b.   Not affected by changes in maternal or fetal positioning
4.   Disadvantages of internal electronic monitoring
     a.   Increased risk of maternal infection
     b.   Insertion of the spiral electrode into the fetal presenting part may cause a laceration or abscess
     c.   Wires may limit maternal movement
     d.   Attention could be focused on the monitor instead of the mother.
     e.   Electrode/catheter cannot be inserted until membranes rupture, cervix dilates to at least 1 cm, and the fetus descends

S. Uterine contractions
1. Phases
   a. Increment: the building-up phase and longest phase
   b. Acme: the peak of the contraction
   c. Decrement: the letting-up phase
2. Duration
   a. Measured from the beginning of one contraction to the end of the same contraction
   b. Averages 30 seconds in early labor and 60 seconds in later labor
3. Frequency
   a. Measured from the beginning of one contraction to the beginning of the next
   b. Contractions average 5 to 30 minutes apart in early labor, increasing to 2 to 3 minutes apart in later labor
4. Intensity
   a. Strength of the contraction during the acme phase is measured with intrauterine catheter or by palpation
   b. Normal resting pressure when using an intrauterine catheter is 10 mm Hg, with an increase to 30 to 50 mm Hg during the acme

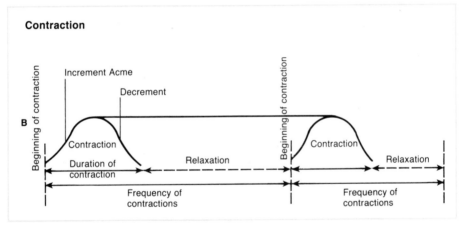

5. Early decelerations of fetal heart rate
   a. Cause: head compression
   b. Shape: uniform, smooth waveform that inversely mirrors the corresponding contraction
   c. Range: within normal range of 120 to 160 beats/minute
   d. Clinical significance: reassuring pattern; not associated with any fetal difficulties
   e. Nursing intervention: none required
6. Late decelerations of fetal heart rate
   a. Cause: uteroplacental insufficiency

Decelerations

**Early
decelerations**

**Late
decelerations**

**Variable
decelerations**

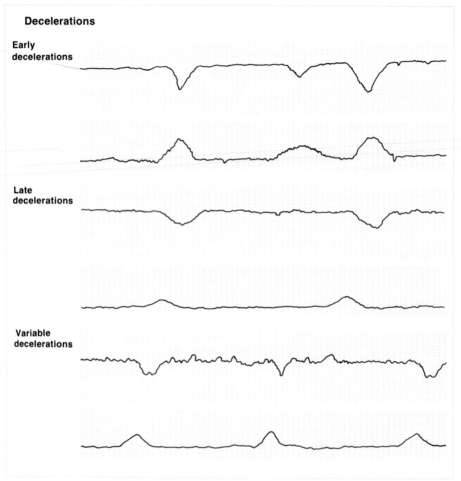

b. Shape: smooth, uniform waveforms that inversely mirror the contractions but are late in their onset

c. Range: usually within the normal range with a high baseline; may drop to below 100 beats/minute when severe

d. Clinical significance: considered an ominous sign if persistent and uncorrected; pattern is associated with decreased Apgar scores, fetal hypoxia, and acidosis

e. Nursing interventions: change maternal position to the left lateral position, increase the primary I.V. flow rate, administer oxygen via face mask following hospital protocol or physician's order (frequently 6 to 8 L/minute), discontinue oxytocin if infusing, assist with fetal blood sampling if ordered

7. Variable decelerations of fetal heart rate
   a. Cause: umbilical cord compression
   b. Shape: vary in onset, occurrence, and waveform
   c. Range: in severe cases, heart rate may decelerate below 70 beats/minute for more than 30 seconds, with a slow return to baseline
   d. Clinical significance: occur in approximately 50% of labors and are usually transient and correctable; occurrences are not associated with low Apgar scores
   e. Nursing interventions: administer oxygen via face mask following hospital protocol or physician's order (frequently 6 to 8 L/minute), continue to monitor
8. Accelerations of fetal heart rate
   a. Cause: normally from fetal movements but also occurs with contractions
   b. Shape: uniform or variable shape
   c. Range: usually above 150 beats/minute
   d. Clinical significance: signifies fetal well-being
   e. Nursing interventions: none required
9. Variability of fetal heart rate
   a. Cause: the normal irregularity of the cardiac rhythm, caused by the continuous interplay of the parasympathetic and sympathetic nervous system
   b. Long-term variability: rhythmic fluctuations and waves; usually three to five times/minute.
   c. Short-term variability: the beat-to-beat changes of heart rate in the baseline. Average beat-to-beat variability is six to 10 beats/minute.
10. Increased variability of fetal heart rate
    a. Cause: early, mild hypoxia and fetal stimulation
    b. Clinical significance: earliest sign of mild fetal hypoxia
    c. Nursing interventions: carefully evaluate FHR tracing for signs of fetal distress
11. Decreased variability of fetal heart rate
    a. Cause: hypoxia, acidosis, central nervous system depressants, medications
    b. Clinical significance: benign when associated with drugs; ominous if caused by hypoxia or associated with late decelerations
    c. Nursing interventions: assist with possible fetal blood sampling and insertion of internal monitor, as ordered
12. Fetal blood sampling
    a. Definition: method of monitoring fetal blood pH when confusing or nonreassuring FHR patterns occur
    b. Procedure: sample is usually taken from the scalp but may also be taken if fetus is breech
    c. Membranes must be ruptured and cervix must be dilated at least 2 to 3 cm; the presenting part must be no higher than −2 station

    d. Results: 7.25 and higher, normal; 7.20 to 7.24, preacidotic; lower than 7.2, serious acidosis

T. Role of the coach during labor and delivery
1. A coach (husband or significant other) is of great value during labor and delivery, especially if the couple has attended prenatal classes together.
2. Benefits and roles of the labor coach include:
    a. Providing emotional support
    b. Providing physical support (back rubs)
    c. Enhancing communication between the mother and staff if necessary (i.e., when there is a language barrier)
    d. Reducing anxiety and pain perception
    e. Aiding in the initiation of bonding with the newborn

U. Obstetrical procedures
1. Episiotomy: an incision of the perineum, performed to enlarge the vaginal outlet
    a. The type of episiotomy depends on the site and direction of incision
    b. Advantages of episiotomy: prevents tearing (laceration) of the perineum; can be repaired more easily than a tear and will heal faster; enlarges the vaginal outlet to facilitate manipulation or use of forceps
    c. Disadvantages of episiotomy: discomfort from episiotomy may interfere with maternal/infant bonding; incision creates a potential site of infection; discomfort may make client hesitant to void and/or have a bowel movement
2. Forceps: double-bladed instrument used in delivery
    a. Commonly used forceps: Kjelland, Elliot, Piper, Tucker-McLean, and Simpson
    b. Types of forceps deliveries: outlet (low) forceps, when the fetal head is visible on the perineum; midforceps, when the fetal head is located at the ischial spines; high forceps, when the vertex is not engaged; this is a very dangerous use of forceps, and is rarely done
    c. Advantages of forceps: shortens the second stage of labor when adverse fetal and maternal conditions exist
    d. Disadvantages of forceps: increased perinatal morbidity and mortality with midforceps delivery; increased neonatal birth trauma and depression; increased incidence of postpartum hemorrhage
3. Cesarean delivery: removal of infant from the uterus via an abdominal incision
    a. Indications include: cephalopelvic disproportion; uterine dysfunction; malposition or malpresentation; previous uterine surgery; complete or partial placenta previa; preexisting medical condition (i.e., diabetes, cardiac disease); prolapsed uterine cord; and fetal distress
    b. Uterine incisions: transverse incision, the most common and preferred due to decreased incidence of peritonitis, decreased postoperative

adhesions and minimal blood loss; or classic (vertical) incision, used when adhesions from previous cesarean exist, when the fetus is in a transverse lie, and with an anteriorly implanted placenta

V. Induction of labor

1. Readiness for induction depends on three factors:
   a. Fetal maturity, as assessed by amniotic fluid studies and serial ultrasound examinations
   b. Cervical readiness, as assessed by cervical dilatation, effacement, consistency, and position
   c. Fetal position

Bishop score for assessing readiness for induction

	Score*				
	0	1	2	3	Subtotals
Dilatation (cm)	0	1–2	3–4	5–6	
Effacement (%)	0–30	40–50	60–70	80	
Station (cm)	–3	–2	–1	+1	
Cervical consistency	Firm	Medium	Soft		
Fetal position	Posterior	Midline	Anterior		
					TOTAL

*Parous woman can be induced at score of 5; nulliparous woman, at score of 7.

2. Indications for induction
   a. Postmaturity (greater than 42 weeks of gestation); placental insufficiency and fetal compromise may exist
   b. Premature rupture of membranes; increased risk of intrauterine infection may exist
   c. Pregnancy-induced hypertension; condition may worsen
   d. Rh isoimmunization; induce to prevent erythroblastosis fetalis
   e. Maternal diabetes; induce to prevent fetal demise from placental insufficiency
   f. Fetal demise
3. Maternal contraindications for induction
   a. Grand multiparity
   b. Placental abnormalities
   c. Previous uterine surgery
   d. Overdistention of the uterus
   e. Structural abnormalities of the vagina, uterus, or pelvis
4. Fetal contraindications for induction
   a. Abnormal fetal lie
   b. Fetal distress
   c. Premature or low-birth-weight fetus
   d. Positive OCT

5. Advantages of induction
   a. Client can be physically and psychologically prepared for labor and delivery
   b. Existing medical condition(s) that could interfere with fetal well-being can be resolved
6. Disadvantages of induction
   a. Possible risk to fetus from increased uterine activity and chance of prematurity
   b. Increased risks to mother due to prolonged labor, cervical laceration, and postpartum hemorrhage
   c. Physical and psychological stress if induction fails
7. Induction via amniotomy: the artificial rupturing of membranes by use of a sterile instrument; under favorable conditions, approximately 80% of women will enter labor within 24 hours
   a. Advantages: facilitates fetal status monitoring via internal scalp electrode, catheter, or scalp blood sampling; facilitates assessment of color and composition of amniotic fluid
   b. Disadvantages: increased risk of infection and prolapsed cord; increased incidence of fetal head compression
   c. Indications for amniotomy: when internal fetal monitoring is desired and use of oxytocin is contraindicated
   d. Contraindications for amniotomy: presenting part is at -2 station or higher; placenta previa; abnormal presenting part; uncertain estimated date of confinement (EDC) and presence of herpesvirus II in vagina
8. Induction via oxytocin infusion: administration of intravenous oxytocin (Pitocin) to augment or stimulate uterine contractions
   a. Advantages of oxytocin infusion: predictability of action; no direct effect on fetus; efficient and effective method of stimulating contractions
   b. Disadvantages of oxytocin infusion: increased risk of tetanic uterine contractions and overstimulation of the uterus, leading to fetal distress and uterine rupture
   c. Indications for oxytocin infusion: prolonged ROM; postmaturity; termination of pregnancy necessary due to adverse maternal or fetal conditions
   d. Contraindications for oxytocin infusion: cephalopelvic disproportion (CPD); fetal distress; previous uterine surgery; overdistended uterus; abnormal fetal presentation
   e. Nursing interventions: assess FHR and contraction pattern by continuous electronic monitoring; stop infusion immediately if signs of fetal distress or tetanic uterine contractions occur; continue interventions discussed in Section V-H

W. Possible complications during labor and delivery

1. Dystocia: difficult labor due to either mechanical and/or functional factors
    a. Mechanical factors (maternal): contracted pelvis and obstructive tumors
    b. Mechanical factors (fetal): malpresentation, malformed fetus
    c. Functional factors: dysfunctional uterine patterns such as hypertonic and hypotonic
2. Premature rupture of membranes (PROM): rupturing of membranes 1 or more hours before the onset of labor
    a. Chorioamnionitis may occur if the latent period (time between ROM and onset of labor) is longer than 24 hours
    b. Signs of chorioamnionitis include fetal tachycardia, maternal fever, foul-smelling amniotic fluid, and uterine tenderness
    d. PROM is associated with malpresentation, incompetent cervix, subclinical infection, advanced maternal age, multiparity, and preterm labor
    e. Fetal/neonatal implications include increased incidence of fetal infection and perinatal mortality
    f. Management includes antibiotic administration if indicated; assessment for signs of infection or fetal distress; possible induction of labor or cesarean delivery if labor does not start within 24 hours
3. Precipitate labor: labor that lasts 3 hours or less; usually caused by lack of maternal tissue resistance to the passage of the fetus
4. Amniotic fluid embolism: escape of amniotic fluid into the maternal circulation via either a defect in the membranes after ROM or partial abruptio placenta
    a. Fetal/neonatal implications: meconium, lanugo, and vernix in fluid may be deposited in the pulmonary arterioles
    b. Clinical manifestations: sudden dyspnea, cyanosis, tachypnea, hemorrhage, chest pain, coughing with pink frothy sputum, increasing restlessness and anxiety, and shock out of proportion to blood loss
    c. Predisposing factors: intrauterine fetal death, high parity, abruptio placenta, oxytocin augmentation, advanced maternal age
    d. Management: administration of oxygen, blood, heparin; insertion of central venous pressure (CVP) line; monitoring of cardiopulmonary status, immediate delivery
5. Prolapsed umbilical cord: descent of the umbilical cord into the vagina before the presenting part
    a. Fetal/neonatal implications: the cord may become compressed between the fetus and maternal cervix or pelvis, thus compromising fetoplacental perfusion; prolapsed umbilical cord is an emergency that requires prompt action to save the fetus
    b. Predisposing factors: abnormal fetal position, multiple gestation, hydramnios, ROM before engagement, and factors that could interfere with fetal descent

      c. Management: positioning of mother in Trendelenburg position; monitoring of FHR; application of saline-soaked sterile dressing over cord; pushing of head upward off cord with sterile gloved hand; immediate delivery

6. Inverted uterus: uterus has turned partially or totally inside out during delivery of the placenta, due to excessive traction on the umbilical cord and/or thin uterine wall

      a. Clinical manifestations: severe uterine pain, hemorrhage, inability to palpate the fundus abdominally, and detection of uterine mass within vaginal canal

      b. Management: restoration of fluid volume; administration of blood; monitoring of vital signs; administration of oxygen via mask, according to hospital policy or doctor's order; immediate manual replacement by doctor; possible emergency hysterectomy

7. Early postpartum hemorrhage: blood loss of 500 ml or more during the first hour after delivery

      a. Causes: uterine atony, lacerations of the vagina and cervix, and hematoma formation. Uterine atony accounts for 80 to 90% of all early hemorrhages

      b. Management: assessment of uterine contraction postdelivery, amount and color of vaginal bleeding, presence of distended bladder, vital signs every 15 minutes until stable; administration of intravenous oxytocin; vaginal examination of possible bleeding sites; uterine massage

      c. Clients at risk: women who deliver a large infant or multiple infants; who received general anesthesia; whose labor was augmented with oxytocin; forceps delivery or rotation; high parity or previous history of hemorrhage; vaginal birth after previous cesarean section (VBAC)

8. Fetal distress: fetal compromise that results in a stressful and potentially lethal condition

      a. Causes: prematurity; uteroplacental insufficiency; congenital malformation; ABO or Rh incompatibility; maternal complications such as diabetes, heart disease, PIH; prolonged labor; postmaturity; oxytocin infusion; and vaginal bleeding

      b. Management: monitor FHR, fetal activity, fetal heart variability; notify physician immediately; prepare for possible placement of internal monitor and fetal scalp pH sampling; position woman on left side; administer oxygen via face mask following hospital protocol or physician's orders (frequently 6 to 8 L/minute); discontinue oxytocin if infusing

9. Lacerations: tears in the perineum, vagina, or cervix due to the stretching of tissues during childbirth. Perineal lacerations are classified as first, second, third, and fourth degree.

      a. First-degree laceration involves the vaginal mucosa and the skin of the perineum to the fourchette

    b. Second-degree laceration involves the vagina, perineal skin, fascia, levator ani muscle, and perineal body

    c. Third-degree laceration involves the entire perineum and the external anal sphincter

    d. Fourth-degree laceration involves the entire perineum, rectal sphincter, and portions of the rectal mucous membrane

10. Disseminated intravascular coagulation (DIC)

    a. Definition: increased production of prothrombin, platelets, and other coagulation factors that leads to widespread thrombi formation throughout the body. Ultimately, the body's clotting factors are expended, leading to hemorrhage

    b. Predisposing factors: abruptio placenta, sepsis, intrauterine fetal death, and amniotic fluid embolism

    c. Clinical manifestations: thrombocytopenia, decreased fibrinogen and platelet count, increased prothrombin time and partial thromboplastin time

    d. Maternal implication: death if hypofibrinogenia does not reverse

    e. Fetal/neonate implications: fetus not directly affected; however, at risk from maternal sepsis, acidosis, and hypotension. Major risk to the fetus/neonate is hypoxia

    f. Management: blood and fibrinogen transfusions; treatment of underlying condition, administration of heparin, and immediate delivery

X. Premature labor: labor that occurs before the end of the 37th week of pregnancy

1. Maternal causes

    a. Cardiovascular and renal disease

    b. Diabetes mellitus

    c. PIH

    d. Infections

    e. Abdominal surgery or trauma

    f. Incompetent cervix

    g. Placental abnormalities

    h. PROM

2. Fetal causes

    a. Infection

    b. Hydramnios

    c. Multiple pregnancy

3. Fetal/neonatal implications: increased morbidity or mortality due to excessive maturational deficiencies (Refer to Section IV-M-12)

4. Management with ritodrine (Yutopar), the most commonly used tocolytic agent

    a. Mechanisms: stimulates β_2 receptors, causing smooth muscle relaxation

    b. Contraindications: gestation less than 20 weeks; cervical dilatations greater than 4 cm; cervical effacement greater than 50%; severe PIH; cardiac disease; and ROM

    c. Maternal side effects: tachycardia, diarrhea, nervousness and tremors, nausea and vomiting, headache, hyper- or hypoglycemia, hypokalemia, pulmonary edema

    d. Fetal side effects: tachycardia, hypoxia, hypoglycemia, and hypocalcemia

    e. Antidote: propranolol (Inderal)

5. Management with magnesium sulfate
   a. Mechanism: prevents reflux of calcium into the myometrial cell, thus maintaining a relaxed uterus
   b. Side effects: magnesium sulfate toxicity is manifested by CNS depression in the mother.

6. Management with terbutaline sulfate (Brethine)
   a. Mechanism: acts as a smooth muscle relaxant
   b. Side effects: maternal and fetal tachycardia, nervousness, headache, and neonatal hypoglycemia

7. Nursing interventions during premature labor
   a. Provide emotional support
   b. Monitor laboratory results
   c. Monitor maternal vital signs and FHR
   d. Monitor status of contractions
   e. Notify physician if maternal pulse exceeds 120 beats/minute and FHR exceeds 180 beats/minute
   f. Position client in left lateral position to increase placental perfusion
   g. Have antidotes readily available
   h. If client is discharged on Ritodrine, review the signs and symptoms she should immediately report and the activity level she should maintain, as ordered by physician.

Y. Optional birthing experiences

1. Birth centers: maternity facilities located in a hospital or separate institution close to a hospital. Such centers provide a warm, homelike environment in which families are required to take more responsibility for the birth experience. Centers are not appropriate for high-risk deliveries; majority of care is provided by nurse-midwives.
2. Home births: controversial option because of inadequate medical back-up
3. Siblings at birth: prenatal education of and active participation by siblings foster the integration of the newborn into the family
4. Optional positioning: alternatives to the lithotomy position include side-lying, squatting, sitting, and semi-Fowler's
5. Leboyer method: a controversial, soothing, tender approach to handling the infant immediately after delivery. Lights are dimmed, noise level diminished. After the cord is clamped, the newborn is gently and slowly placed in a warm bath.

Points to Remember

The process of labor and delivery marks the ultimate crisis for the pregnant woman, her fetus, and family.

To ensure early identification of problems, the nurse must understand fetal monitor strip interpretations.

A woman's perception of her labor and delivery experience depends on numerous factors.

A woman may feel that she has failed labor if she undergoes a cesarean section delivery.

Glossary

Dilatation—widening of the external cervical os

Effacement—thinning and shortening of the cervix

Molding—shaping of the fetal head by overlapping of the sutures; helps the head conform to the birth canal

Station—Relationship of the presenting part to the ischial spines

Obstetrical Analgesia and Anesthesia

Learning Objectives

After studying this section, the reader should be able to:

- Discuss current theories of pain.

- Identify potential sources of pain during labor and delivery.

- Describe pharmacologic and nonpharmacologic methods of pain relief during labor and delivery.

- Discuss the nurse's role in caring for a client who has received analgesics and/or anesthesia during labor and delivery.

- Describe potential maternal, fetal, and neonatal side effects of pharmacologic measures used during labor and delivery.

VI. Obstetrical Analgesia and Anesthesia

A. Pain perception

1. Theories of pain
   a. Specificity: a specific pain system carries messages from pain receptors in the body to a pain center in the brain
   b. Pattern: particular networks of nerve impulses are produced by sensory input at the dorsal horn cells. Pain results when the output of these cells exceeds a critical level.
   c. Gate control: local physical stimulation can balance the pain stimuli by closing down a hypothetical "gate" in the spinal cord that blocks pain signals from reaching the brain
2. Sources of pain during labor
   a. Dilatation and stretching of the cervix
   b. Emotional tension
   c. Hypoxia of the uterine muscle cells during a contraction
   d. Stretching of the lower uterine segment
   e. Pressure by the presenting part on adjacent structures (bowel, bladder)
   f. Distention of the vagina and perineum
3. Factors affecting pain perception
   a. Cultural background: individuals tend to react to pain in ways that are acceptable in their individual culture
   b. Personal significance: how an individual regards pain is closely aligned with self-concept
   c. Fatigue and sleep deprivation: a tired individual has less energy and cannot focus on such strategies as distraction
   d. Attention and distractions: preoccupation with another activity (breathing techniques) lessens pain perception

B. Pain relief during labor and delivery: nonpharmacologic measures

1. Effleurage: light abdominal stroking with the fingertips in a circular motion. Effective for mild to moderate discomfort
2. Distraction: diversion of attention from discomfort during early labor by reading, playing games, and recalling pleasant experiences
3. Controlled breathing: Lamaze breathing consists of three patterns of chest breathing
   a. Slow chest: inhaling through nose and exhaling through the mouth or nose six to nine times/minute
   b. Accelerated/decelerated: as contractions become more intense, air is inhaled through the nose and exhaled through the mouth
   c. Pant-blow: during transitional phase, client takes rapid, shallow breaths throughout the contraction, breathing only through the mouth

C. Pain relief during labor and delivery: analgesic agents

1. Narcotics
   a. The most frequently used drug is meperidine (Demerol)
   b. Common maternal side effects are respiratory depression, nausea and vomiting, drowsiness, and transient hypotension.
   c. Common fetal/neonatal side effects are neonatal respiratory depression if medication is given within 2 hours of delivery, hypotonia, and lethargy
2. Sedatives
   a. Barbiturates are commonly used in false labor or in early prodromal labor
   b. Secobarbital (Seconal) and pentobarbital sodium (Nembutal) are commonly used barbiturates

D. Pain relief during labor and delivery: anesthetic agents

1. General: administered intravenously or by inhalation, resulting in unconsciousness
   a. Inhalation anesthetics: nitrous oxide, Penthrane, and Fluothane
   b. Intravenous anesthetics: pentothal and ketamine
   c. Maternal complications: vomiting and aspiration, increased uterine relaxation, possibly leading to postpartum uterine atony
   d. Fetal/neonatal complications: respiratory depression, hypotonia, and lethargy
2. Regional: local anesthetics injected to block pain neuropathways that pass from the uterus to the spinal cord via sympathetic nerves
   a. Lumbar epidural anesthesia: the injection of medication into the epidural space in the lumbar region. The epidural leaves the client awake and cooperative; it provides analgesia for the first and second stages and anesthesia for delivery, without direct adverse effects on fetus. Disadvantages of epidural: hypotension; decreased urge to push; risk of dural puncture and increased need for forceps
   b. Spinal: the injection of medication into the cerebrospinal fluid in the spinal canal; has low incidence of side effects and rapid onset, but causes postspinal headache, increased incidence and degree of hypotension, and urinary retention
   c. Local infiltration: the injection of anesthesia into the nerves of the perineum; it is simple to administer and has no side effects on fetus but does not provide relief from discomfort during labor, only at delivery
   d. Pudendal block: the blockage of the pudendal nerve; it is simple, safe, and does not depress the fetus but does not relieve discomfort from uterine contractions, only discomfort from perineal distention

e. Paracervical: the blockage of nerves in the peridural space at the sacral hiatus; it leaves the client awake, has little effect on fetus, provides analgesia for the first and second stages of labor and anesthesia for delivery; it also causes increased incidence of hypotension, increased use of forceps, fetal bradycardia, and hematomas

3. Nursing interventions during the administration of analgesic and anesthetic agents: the nurse must know each type of anesthesia and analgesia used in obstetrics to:
   a. Allay the client's fears and anxieties about medication
   b. Help the anesthesiologist and obstetrician
   c. Be familiar with possible maternal and fetal side effects of the various medications
   d. Take swift action if adverse reaction(s) occur
   e. Answer the client's questions

Points to Remember

Nurses must be familiar enough with anesthetic and analgesic agents to answer a client's questions, assist the anesthesiologist and obstetrician, and identify adverse maternal, fetal, and neonatal effects quickly.

Pain perception is an individualized reaction that is affected by physical, sociocultural, and psychological factors.

The client's blood pressure must be monitored following epidural, spinal, paracervical, and regional anesthesia.

The client's understanding of the potential sources of pain during labor and delivery can alleviate anxiety.

Glossary

Analgesic—a pharmacologic agent that relieves pain without causing unconsciousness

Anesthesia—the use of pharmacologic agents to produce partial or total loss of sensation with or without loss of consciousness

General anesthesia—use of pharmacologic agents to produce loss of consciousness, progressive central nervous system depression, and complete loss of sensation

Local anesthesia—blockage of sensory nerve pathways at the organ level, producing loss of sensation only in that organ

Regional anesthesia—blockage of large sensory nerve pathways in an organ and its surrounding tissue, producing loss of sensation in that organ and in the surrounding region

The Postpartum Client

Learning Objectives

After studying this section, the reader should be able to:

● Describe the normal physiologic changes that occur during the postpartum period.

● Trace the course of psychological adjustment during the postpartum period.

● Identify the points that should be included in a postpartum teaching plan.

● Identify the needs of the mother and her family in adjusting to the new family member.

VII. The Postpartum Client

A. Physiologic changes after pregnancy

1. Vascular system
   a. Decreased blood volume with increased hematocrit after vaginal delivery
   b. Extensive activation of blood clotting factors
   c. Return of blood volume to prenatal levels within 3 weeks
2. Reproductive system
   a. Rapid uterine involution
   b. Cessation of progesterone production until first ovulation
   c. Permanent alteration of cervical external os shape from a circle to a jagged slit
   d. Endometrial regeneration by 6 weeks postdelivery
3. Gastrointestinal system
   a. Delayed bowel movement from decreased intestinal muscle tone, perineal discomfort, and fear
   b. Increased thirst from fluids lost during labor and delivery
   c. Increased hunger after labor and delivery
4. Urinary tract
   a. Increased urine output during first 24 hours after delivery from puerperal diuresis
   b. Increased bladder capacity
   c. Proteinuria from the catalytic process of involution in 50% of women
   d. Decreased bladder-filling sensation from swelling and bruising of tissues
   e. Return of dilated ureters and renal pelvis to prepregnancy size by 6 weeks
5. Endocrine system
   a. Increased thyroid function
   b. Increased production of anterior pituitary gonadotropic hormones
   c. Decreased production of estrogen, aldosterone, progesterone, hCG, corticoids, and 17-ketosteroids

B. Postpartum care: nursing interventions

1. Vital signs
   a. Vital signs should be monitored every 4 hours for the first 24 hours and then every shift thereafter
   b. Client's temperature may be elevated to 100.4°F. (38°C.) from dehydration and exertion of labor
   c. Blood pressure is usually normotensive within 24 hours of delivery
   d. Bradycardia of 50 to 70 beats/minute is common during the first 6 to 10 days after delivery, due to decreased cardiac strain, decreased stroke volume, and decrease in the vascular bed
   e. Normal respiratory rate returns after delivery

2. Fundus: the uppermost portion of the uterus
   a. The nurse should assess the tone and location of the fundus on every shift to assess the involution process
   b. The fundus is usually midway between the umbilicus and symphysis 1 to 2 hours after delivery
   c. The fundus is usually 1 cm above or at the level of the umbilicus 12 hours postdelivery
   d. The fundus is approximately 3 cm below the umbilicus by the third day postdelivery
   e. The fundus will continue to descend at approximately 1 cm/day until it is not palpable above the symphysis at 9 days postdelivery
   f. The uterus returns to its prepregnancy size 5 to 6 weeks postdelivery. Decrease in size is not from a decrease in the number of cells, but from a decrease in the size of the individual cells
   g. A distended bladder can impede the downward descent of the uterus by pushing it upward and possibly to the side
   h. The involuting uterus should be at the midline
   i. The fundus should feel firm to the touch
   j. A firm uterus helps control postpartum hemorrhage by clamping down on uterine blood vessels
   k. A boggy (soft) fundus should be massaged gently; if the fundus does not respond, a firmer touch should be used
   l. The uterus may relax if overstimulated
   m. The client may need oxytocic medication such as oxytocin (Pitocin), ergonovine maleate (Ergotrate Maleate), or methylergonovine maleate (Methergine) to maintain uterine firmness
   n. Multiparas are more prone to "after-pains" from uterine contractions; "after-pains" generally last 2 to 3 days and may be intensified by breastfeeding

3. Lochia
   a. The nurse should assess the lochia during every shift, noting the color, amount, odor, and consistency
   b. The vaginal discharge for the first 3 days after delivery is called lochia rubra; it has a fleshy odor and is bloody with small clots
   c. Lochia serosa refers to the vaginal discharge during days 4 to 9; it is pinkish or brown with a serosanguineous consistency and fleshy odor
   d. Lochia alba is a yellow to white discharge that usually begins 10 days or so after delivery
   e. Lochia alba may last from 2 to 6 weeks after delivery
   f. Foul-smelling lochia may indicate an infection
   g. Continuous seepage of bright red blood may indicate a cervical or vaginal laceration. Additional evaluation is necessary
   h. A heavier flow of lochia may occur when the client first rises from bed, from pooling of the lochia in the vagina
   i. The presence of numerous large clots should be evaluated further; they may interfere with the involution process

    j. Breastfeeding and exertion may increase lochial flow

    k. Lochial discharge may be decreased after a cesarean delivery

    l. Lochia may be scant but should never be absent; this may indicate a postpartum infection

    m. Lochia that saturates a sanitary pad within 45 minutes usually indicates an abnormally heavy flow

4. Breasts

    a. The nurse should assess the size and shape of the breasts on every shift, noting reddened areas, tenderness, or engorgement

    b. The nurse should check the nipples for cracking, fissures, and/or soreness

    c. The client should wear a support bra to maintain shape and enhance comfort

5. Elimination

    a. The client should void within the first 6 hours after delivery

    b. The nurse should assess for a distended bladder within the first few hours after delivery; a distended bladder can interfere with uterine involution

    c. The client may use pain medication before urination and/or pour warm water over the perineum to eliminate the fear of pain

    d. The client who cannot void may have to be catheterized

    e. The client should be encouraged to have a bowel movement within a day or two after delivery to avoid constipation

    f. The nurse should encourage increased fluid and roughage intake and alleviate maternal anxieties regarding pain and damage to episiotomy

    g. The client may require laxatives, stool softeners, suppositories, or enemas

    h. A client with a fourth-degree laceration should never be given anything rectally

6. Episiotomy

    a. The episiotomy should be assessed every shift to evaluate the healing process

    b. The edges of an episiotomy are usually sealed 24 hours postdelivery

    c. The episiotomy should be assessed for erythema, intactness of stitches, edema, and any odor or drainage

    d. The client can be positioned on the same side that her mediolateral episiotomy was performed on to provide better visibility and less discomfort

    e. A woman with a midline episiotomy may be positioned either on her side or on her back during assessment

    f. The rectal area should be assessed for the presence of hemorrhoids; note the number and appearance

7. Medications commonly used in the postpartum client for discomfort from engorged breasts, episiotomy, uterine contractions, incisional pain
   a. Analgesics such as propoxyphene hydrochloride (Darvocet-N); acetaminophen; aspirin; oxycodone hydrochloride (Perocet); and caffeine, butalbital (Fiorinal), and codeine
   b. Stool softeners and laxatives such as docusate calcium (Surfak), docusate sodium (Colace), and magnesium salts (Milk of Magnesia)
   c. Prenatal vitamins
   d. Oxytocic agents such as methylergonovine maleate (Methergine), oxytocin (Pitocin), and ergonovine maleate (Ergotrate Maleate) to prevent or treat postpartum hemorrhage
   e. Lactation supressors such as bromocriptine mesylate (Parlodel) and, less frequently, chlorotrianisene (Tace) and testosterone enanthate, estradiolevalerate, and chlorobutanol (Deladumone)

C. **Psychological adjustment during the postpartum period, as identified by Reva Rubin**
   1. "Taking-in" phase: first 1 to 2 days after delivery
      a. Mother is passive and dependent
      b. Mother directs energy towards herself instead of her infant
      c. Mother may relive her labor and delivery to integrate the process into her life
      d. Mother may find decision-making difficult
   2. "Taking-hold" phase
      a. Mother's energy level increases
      b. Mother demonstrates independence and initiation of self-care activities
      c. Mother accepts increasing responsibility for her newborn
      d. Mother may be receptive to infant care and self-care education
      e. Mother may verbalize lack of confidence in caring for infant
   3. "Letting-go" phase
      a. A time for reorganization of family ties
      b. A time for mother to assume responsibility for her dependent newborn
      c. A time to recognize infant as separate from self and to relinquish fantasized infant
      d. A time when feelings of depression are common
   4. The above phases are not meant to be strict guidelines for the assessment of maternal behavior. Instead, they can help the nurse understand maternal behavior.

D. **Postpartum teaching: maternal self-care guidelines**
   1. Personal hygiene
      a. Perineal pads should be changed frequently, removing from front to back
      b. Lochia with a foul smell, heavy flow, and/or clots should be reported immediately

    c. A sitz bath should be used three to four times a day

    d. Daily showers can relieve the discomfort of normal postpartum diaphoresis

2. Sexual activity

    a. Most couples resume sexual activity within 3 to 4 weeks after delivery, thus necessitating the need to review contraception

    b. Breast feeding is not a reliable form of contraception

    c. Vaginal lubrication may be diminished for up to 6 months, due to steroid depletion; encourage use of a water-based lubricant such as K-Y Jelly

    d. The woman may experience decreased intensity and rapidity of sexual response; this is a normal reaction for approximately 3 months after delivery

    e. Kegel exercises can help strengthen pubococcygeal muscles

    f. 50% of bottle-feeding mothers ovulate during the first cycle postdelivery; 80% of breastfeeding mothers have several anovulatory cycles before ovulating

3. Weight loss

    a. Mothers usually lose 10 to 12 lbs after delivery; diuresis causes an additional loss of 5 lbs during the early puerperium period

    b. Mothers can expect to return to their prepregnancy weight by approximately 6 to 8 weeks after delivery *if* weight gain during pregnancy averaged 25 to 30 lbs

4. Activity and exercise

    a. Increased abdominal muscle tone occurs within 2 to 3 months after delivery

    b. Exercises can begin when the mother's condition permits

    c. An increase in the amount of lochia or return to lochia rubra may indicate excessive activity. Mother should sit down for approximately 30 minutes with her legs elevated; if excessive vaginal discharge persists, notify the physician

    d. Mother should be assisted out of bed the first several times after delivery; there is an increased incidence of dizziness and fainting from medications, blood loss, and decreased food intake

5. Nutrition

    a. Postpartum mothers should increase protein and caloric intake to restore body tissues

    b. Breastfeeding mothers should increase caloric intake by 200 kcal over the pregnancy requirement of 2,400 kcal

    c. Postpartum mothers will experience increased thirst because of postpartum diuresis

6. Comfort measures
   a. For the perineal area: ice packs (for the first 8 to 12 hours to minimize edema); squirt peri bottles; sitz baths; anesthetic sprays, creams, and pads (witch hazel pads); medications
   b. For engorged breasts: tight supportive bra or binder; ice packs; medications; frequent meals if breastfeeding; warm compresses and/or manual expression of milk from engorged breasts if breastfeeding

E. **Postpartum teaching: newborn care guidelines for parents**
   1. Cord care
      a. Wipe umbilical cord with alcohol, especially around the base, at every diaper change
      b. Report promptly any odor, discharge, or signs of skin irritation around the cord
      c. Fold the diaper below the cord until the cord falls off, at 7 to 10 days of life
   2. Circumcision
      a. Cleanse penis gently with water and apply fresh petrolatum gauze with each diaper change
      b. Do not remove yellow exudate that covers glans about 24 hours after circumcision; this discharge is part of normal healing
      c. Report promptly foul-smelling, purulent exudate
      d. Loosen petrolatum gauze stuck to penis easily and gently by pouring warm water over area
      e. Apply the diaper loosely until the circumcision heals, in approximately 5 days
   3. Uncircumcised penis
      a. Do not retract the foreskin of the penis when washing the newborn, because the foreskin is adhered to the glans
      b. Understand that natural loosening of the foreskin begins at birth; however, it is retractable in only 50% of males age 1
   4. Thermometer use at home
      a. Insert ½" of lubricated thermometer into rectum for 4 to 5 minutes; carefully place axillary thermometer under arm and hold in place 10 minutes
      b. Learn how to read and shake down a thermometer before infant is discharged from hospital
      c. Advise use of plastic temperature strips for parents who cannot read a glass thermometer
   5. Car seat: note that a car seat is legally required in some states
   6. Diapering
      a. Discuss disposable diapers vs. cloth diapers
      b. Change diapers before and after every feeding
      c. Avoid diaper rash by frequent diaper changes and thorough cleansing and drying of the skin and skin folds

    d. Expose the infant's buttocks to the air and light several times a day for approximately 20 minutes to treat diaper rash; an ointment can be applied to area to decrease contact of the skin with urine and feces

    e. Do not use ointments and powders together; they will cake on the skin and further irritate it

7. Cleansing

    a. Give infant sponge baths until the cord falls off; the child can then be washed in a tub containing 3" to 4" of warm water

    b. Place a wash cloth on the bottom of the tub or sink to prevent slipping

    c. Avoid use of perfumed or deodorant soap

    d. Organize supplies before bath to avoid interruptions

    e. Avoid drafts

    f. Clean the eye from inner to outer canthus with plain water

    g. Vary frequency of bathing with weather; a bath every other day during winter is sufficient

8. Clothing

    a. Dress infant as heavily or lightly as parents would dress themselves

    b. Provide infant with a hat to avoid drafts and minimize heat loss through the scalp while outdoors

9. Formula preparation and feeding

    a. Follow instructions given by pediatrician

    b. Investigate various forms of formula available (ready-to-feed, concentrated, and powder) and preparation methods

    c. Feed baby in an upright position and keep the nipple full of formula to minimize the amount of air swallowed while bottle feeding

    d. Hold infant upright against the shoulder for optimal burping

    e. Avoid holding the infant across the lap while burping; it may bring up milk along with the air

    f. Avoid holding the infant in a sitting position; it may be ineffective because the air cannot easily exit the stomach

    g. Recognize that if an infant has not burped after 3 minutes of gentle patting and rubbing, he/she may not need to burp

    h. Burp newborns after each ounce of formula, and more frequently if infant spits up

10. Handling

    a. Infants have an inborn fear of falling and become upset if left unsupported or if their position is abruptly changed

    b. Infants should not be startled; talk to and touch gently before picking up

    c. The newborn's head must be supported since he/she cannot control it

11. Signs of illness to report to pediatrician

    a. Temperature greater than 101° F. (38.4° C.) or below 97° F. (36.1° C.)

    b. Projectile vomiting

    c. Lethargy

    d. Cyanosis

      e. Change in normal feeding pattern

      f. Change in normal elimination pattern

12. Prevention of illness

      a. Avoidance of ill individuals, crowds

      b. Adequate covering

13. Elimination

      a. Newborns usually have six to eight wet diapers/day

      b. Newborns usually have two to three stools/day, breastfed babies have stools more frequently

      c. The first stool is called meconium; it is an odorless, dark-green, thick substance containing bile, fetal epithelial cells, and hair

      d. Transitional stools occur approximately 2 to 3 days after ingestion of milk; they are greenish-brown and less thick then meconium.

      e. The stool changes to a pasty, yellow, pungent stool (bottle-fed) or to a sweet-smelling loose yellow stool (breast-fed) by the fourth day

14. Breastfeeding

      a. The nipples and areolae should be washed with plain warm water after each feeding and allowed to air dry during the first 2 to 3 weeks to prevent nipple soreness. After that, daily washing is adequate for cleanliness.

      b. Soap should be avoided; it may cause drying and cracking of the nipples and leave an undesirable taste

      c. Creams that do not contain alcohol may be applied to the nipple and areola to prevent drying and cracking

      d. A well-fitted nursing bra provides support and contains flaps that can be loosened easily before feeding

      e. A common occurrence in the early weeks of breastfeeding is leakage of milk and possible staining of clothing. Breast pads can be placed in the bra to avoid staining, but wet pads must be changed promptly to avoid skin breakdown

      f. The most common position for breastfeeding is the cradle position, with the mother seated comfortably and pillows placed for maternal and infant comfort

      g. Other possible positions are the football hold, side-lying position, and the Australian or back-lying position

      h. The mother should initiate breastfeeding as soon as possible after delivery and should then feed the infant on demand

      i. 90% of breast milk will be emptied from the breasts within the first 5 to 7 minutes of feeding

      j. The infants's mouth should be positioned slightly differently at each feeding to reduce irritation at one site

      k. Infants should be burped between breasts

      l. Breast milk can be removed from the breast via manual expression or with a breast pump

      m. Expressed breast milk can be placed into a sterile bottle and stored in the refrigerator for 24 hours

   n. Expressed breast milk can be frozen for up to 4 months
   o. Breastfeeding mothers should drink at least four 8-oz glasses of fluid/day
   p. No specific food restrictions for the breastfeeding mother but she must know that ingested substances (caffeine, alcohol, and medications) can pass into her milk. Common sense, personal tolerance, and moderation should prevail. If the infant appears irritable, gassy, or has diarrhea after a certain food is eaten by the mother, that food should be eliminated from the diet
   q. The mother should insert her little finger into the corner of the baby's mouth to break the suction when separating the baby from the nipple
   r. Breastfeeding mothers should consult their pediatricians before taking medication
   s. All mothers should be given the name and phone number of a breastfeeding support group before discharge from the hospital
   t. Engorged breasts can be emptied via hand pump

F. Postpartum complications
   1. Mastitis: inflammation of the breast, seen primarily in breastfeeding mothers
      a. Causative organism: *Staphylococcus aureus* from the newborn's throat or nose, from hospital personnel or from the mother
      b. Clinical manifestations: temperature; a reddened, warm, tender breast usually appearing 2 to 4 weeks after delivery. Mastitis is usually unilateral and breast milk may become scant
      c. Prevention: frequent breastfeeding; good handwashing; manual release of blocked milk ducts
      d. Management: administration of antibiotics and analgesics, local heat; opinions vary concerning continuation or stoppage of breastfeeding during the acute phase
   2. Late postpartum hemorrhage: blood loss greater than 500 ml, occurring later than 24 hours after delivery. The hemorrhage may not occur until 5 to 15 days after delivery
      a. Predisposing factors: delivery of a large infant; hydramnios; dystocia; grand multiparity; trauma during delivery
      b. Etiology: uterine atony, incomplete placental separation, laceration of the birth canal, and retained placental fragments
      c. Management: careful assessment of uterine tone; assessment of color, amount, and consistency of lochia; vital signs; maintenance of a pad count; administration of oxytocics
   3. Subinvolution of the uterus: failure of the uterus to return to its normal size after childbirth
      a. Predisposing factors: retained placental fragments and infection
      b. Clinical manifestations: displacement of the uterus in the abdominal cavity; persistent lochia rubra, leukorrhea, and backache

    c. Management: diagnosis is usually made at the post-partum checkup, 4 to 6 weeks after delivery. Treatment includes medication (oxytocins and antibiotics) and a possible dilatation and curretage

4. Puerperal psychiatric disorders: depression, mania, and schizophrenia, occurring in approximately 1 to 2% of all normal childbirths

    a. Clinical manifestations of depression include suicidal thinking, feelings of failure and exhaustion which may last up to several months; the most common disorder; peaks approximately 6 weeks postdelivery

    b. Management of depression: psychotherapy and medications (tranquilizer with a prominent stimulating effect)

    c. Clinical manifestations of a manic reaction include agitation and excitement, which may last 1 to 3 weeks; manic reactions may occur 1 to 2 weeks after delivery, sometimes after a brief period of depression

    d. Management of manic reactions: psychotherapy and medications (tranquilizer with a prominent sedative effect)

    e. Clinical manifestations of schizophrenia include delusional thinking, gross distortion of reality, flight of ideas, and possible rejection of the husband and/or infant; may appear by the 10th day postdelivery

    f. Management of schizophrenia: medication (phenothiazine type of tranquilizer), psychotherapy, and possible hospitalization

5. Hematoma: collection of blood (25 to 500 ml) in the soft tissue; the vulva and vagina are the most common sites

    a. Etiology: vascular injury in childbirth, occurring during a spontaneous or assisted delivery

    b. Clinical manifestations: severe vulvar pain; unilateral purplish discoloration of the perineum and buttocks, all of which are firm and tender to the touch; feeling of fullness in the vagina

    c. Management: application of small ice packs and surgical evacuation

6. Puerperal infections: a postpartum infection of the reproductive tract that may remain localized (endometritis, salpingitis) or extend to other parts of the body (peritonitis, pelvic cellulitis)

    a. Etiology: introduction of vaginal microorganisms into the sterile uterine cavity via PROM, operative incisions, hematomas, damaged tissues, and lapses in aseptic technique

    b. Clinical manifestations, depending on the site and extent of infectious process: foul-smelling lochia; lethargy; abdominal pain; subinvolution of the uterus; sustained fever of 100.4° F. (38° C.) or higher

    c. Management: antibiotic therapy; sitz baths; positioning to enhance drainage; maintenance of fluid and electrolyte balance; monitoring of vital signs and symptoms

    d. Note: because a large percentage of postpartum morbidity is from infection, the Joint Committee on Maternal Welfare issued the following definition of puerperal morbidity: "Temperature of 100.4° F. (38° C.) or above, the temperature to occur on any two of the first 10 postpartum days, exclusive of the first 24 hours and to be taken by mouth by a standard technique at least four times a day."

G. Impact of newborn upon family
1. Siblings
   a. Siblings normally dislike the idea of sharing parents with the newborn
   b. Reactions of sibling(s) will depend on their age, presence of other siblings, and amount of preparation
   c. Regression is a normal reaction to newborn
2. Paternal reaction
   a. Fathers as well as mothers need to discuss the labor and delivery experience to integrate it into life experiences
   b. Father may feel left out when attention is given to newborn and mother
   c. Fathers usually have less experience and knowledge regarding infant care; they need to be involved in teaching plan
3. Mother-father relationship
   a. Newborn can strain marital relationship because of the large amount of time and effort devoted to caring for him/her
   b. Father may be jealous of mother-infant relationship
   c. Babysitting arrangements should be made to allow private time for the mother and father

H. The Client with Acquired-immune deficiency syndrome (AIDS)
1. AIDS: The Centers for Disease Control (CDC) defines AIDS as a "reliably diagnosed disease which is moderately indicative of an underlying cellular immunodeficiency in a person who has had no known underlying cause of reduced resistance reported to be associated with that disease"
   a. Individuals at risk: women who are steady sexual partners of men in the AIDS high-risk group (hemophiliacs, intravenous drug abusers, homosexual or bisexual men, and Haitians)
   b. Pathophysiology: immunodeficient state allows opportunistic infections to attack the body
   c. Management: maintain strict blood and secretion precautions; wear disposable gloves and plastic apron when in direct contact with the client's blood or body fluids (i.e., lab specimens, dressings, excretions, linen, trash, amniotic fluid, and sanitary pads); dispose of contaminated needles and syringes in a puncture-resistant receptacle in the client's room; double-bag trash and linen before removal from room; place lab specimens in a plastic bag before removal from room
   d. Psychosocial considerations: many psychological implications emerge from the probable low survival rate of the mother and her child. Direct mother-infant contact should not be avoided unless there are open skin lesions. A private room is not always necessary, though strict isolation is necessary if there are open lesions, copious secretions and/or blood, or if the client has tuberculosis

Points to Remember

Nursing care during the postpartum period must include the entire family.

Subinvolution of the uterus can lead to a postpartum hemorrhage.

The postpartum period is marked by complex psychological and physiological adjustments.

The physical care a woman receives during the postpartum period can affect her physical and emotional health for the rest of her life.

Glossary

Involution—reduction of uterine size after delivery, which can take up to 6 weeks

Lochia—vaginal discharge after delivery due to the sloughing of the uterine decidua

Multipara—a woman who has delivered at least one viable fetus

Nullipara—a woman who has never delivered a viable fetus

Puerperium (postpartum)—the interval between delivery and 6 weeks after delivery

The Newborn

Learning Objectives

After studying this section, the reader should be able to:

- Describe the normal physical characteristics of the newborn.

- Describe factors to be included in a gestational age assessment.

- Describe the normal neurological characteristics of the newborn.

- Explain how to perform newborn care.

- Differentiate between the advantages of breastfeeding and bottle feeding.

- Identify potential complications in high-risk newborns.

VIII. The Newborn

A. Care of the newborn in the delivery room

1. Apgar score
    a. A five-part scoring method used to evaluate the newborn at 1 and 5 minutes of age
    b. A score of 8 to 10 indicates the newborn is in no apparent distress; a score below 8 indicates resuscitative measures may be needed

SIGN	0	1	2
Heart rate	Absent	Less than 100	Greater than 100
Respiratory effort	Absent	Slow, irregular	Good crying
Muscle tone	Flaccid	Some flexion of extremities	Active motion
Reflex irritability	None	Grimace	Vigorous cry
Color	Pale, blue	Body pink, blue extremities	Completely pink

2. Identification
    a. To ensure proper identification, footprints of newborn are taken after delivery and kept on a record that includes the mother's fingerprint.
    b. Identification bands with matching numbers are applied to both mother and infant before they leave the delivery room; two bands are placed on the newborn and one on the mother
3. Nurses' responsibilities in the delivery room
    a. Ensure proper airway in infant via suctioning; administer oxygen as needed.
    b. Dry and place infant under warmer with head lower than trunk to promote drainage of secretions
    c. Assess infant for gross abnormalities and/or clinical manifestations of suspected abnormalities
    d. Continue to assess infant using five parts of Apgar score even after 5-minute score is received
    e. Obtain clear footprints and fingerprints from infant
    f. Apply identification bands to mother and infant
    g. Observe infant for voiding and/or meconium
    h. Apply cord clamp and monitor infant for abnormal bleeding from cord
    i. Facilitate bonding between mother and infant

B. Admission to the nursery

1. Physical examination and assessment
    a. Assessment of the newborn is an ongoing process
    b. Physical examination should be performed following guidelines in previous section.

2. Vital signs
   a. The first temperature is taken rectally to check for rectal patency. Continued use of the rectal site is not recommended because of possible rectal mucosa damage. Because of a delay in adjusting to extrauterine existence, temperature at birth may be 96.8° F. (36° C.) but should stabilize within 8 to 12 hours at approximately 98.2° F. (36.8° C.)
   b. The apical pulse should be taken for 60 seconds; normal rate is 120 to 160 beats/min.
   c. Respirations should be counted with a stethoscope for 60 seconds; normal rate is 30 to 60 breaths/min.
3. Vital statistics
   a. Length: average is 45.8 to 52.3 cm (18" to 20.5")
   b. Head circumference: average is 33 to 35 cm (13" to 14")
   c. Chest circumference: average is 32 cm (12.5")
4. Medications
   a. AquaMEPHYTON (Vitamin K) is administered prophylactically to prevent a transient deficiency of coagulation factors II, VII, IX, X
   b. Prophylactic eye treatment for *Neisseria gonorrhoeae* is legally required. Commonly used medications are silver nitrate (1%) and erythromycin ointment

C. Adaptation to extrauterine life

1. Cardiovascular system: with the first breath, the newborn's lungs expand, thus decreasing the pulmonary vascular resistance. Clamping the cord increases systemic vascular resistance and left atrial pressure. Major changes that occur as the newborn adapts to extrauterine life include:
   a. Functional closure of the foramen ovale from changing atrial pressures; anatomic closure may take from several weeks to a year
   b. Constriction of the ductus arteriosus as the result of increasing pO_2. Functional closure occurs within 15 minutes after birth, fibrosis within 3 weeks. The ductus arteriosus eventually occludes and becomes a ligament
   c. Immediate closure of the umbilical vein, arteries, and ductus venosus from the clamping and severing of the umbilical cord. Anatomic fibrosis occurs within 3 to 7 days, and the structures are eventually converted into ligaments
2. Respiratory system
   a. The initial breath is a reflex triggered in response to chilling, noise, light, or pressure changes
   b. Air immediately replaces the fluid that filled the lungs before birth. Approximately 7 to 42 ml of amniotic fluid is squeezed or drained from the lungs during a vaginal delivery. Other lung fluid crosses the alveolar membrane into the capillaries. Retention of fluid greatly impedes normal respiratory adjustment.

3. Renal system
   a. Renal function does not fully mature until after the first year of life. As a result, the neonate has a minimal range of chemical balance and safety.
   b. Decreased ability to excrete drugs and excessive fluid loss can rapidly lead to acidosis and fluid imbalances
4. Gastrointestinal system
   a. Bacteria are not normally present in the newborn's gastrointestinal tract
   b. Bowel sounds can be heard 1 hour after birth
   c. Uncoordinated peristaltic activity in the esophagus exists for the first few days of life
   d. Newborn has a limited ability to digest fats because of absence of amylase and lipase at birth
   e. The lower intestine contains meconium at birth; the first meconium is sterile, greenish black, and viscous, and usually passes within the first 24 hours after delivery
5. Thermogenesis
   a. Normal neonates can produce sufficient heat in an optimal thermal environment
   b. Rapid heat loss may occur in a suboptimal thermal environment via conduction, convection, radiation, and evaporation
6. Immunological system
   a. IgG: a placentally transferred immunoglobin that provides the neonate with antibodies to bacterial and viral agents. IgG can be detected in the fetus at the third month of gestation. The neonate first synthesizes its own IgG during the first 3 months of life, thus compensating for concurrent catabolism of maternal antibodies
   b. IgM: the fetus synthesizes IgM by the 20th week of gestation. IgM does not cross the placenta. Increased levels of IgM in the neonate indicates a nonspecific infection
   c. IgA: not detectable at birth; does not cross the placenta. Secretory IgA is found in colostrum and breast milk; it limits bacterial growth in the gastrointestinal tract
7. Hematopoietic system
   a. Blood volume of term neonate: approximately 80 to 85 ml/kg of body weight
   b. Hemoglobin: 15 to 20 g/dL
   c. Hematocrit: 43% to 61%
   d. Red blood cells: 5 million to 7.5 million/mm^3
   e. White blood cells: 10,000 to 30,000/mm^3
   f. Neutrophils: 40% to 80%
   g. Eosinophils: 2% to 3%
   h. Lymphocytes: 30% to 31%
   i. Monocytes: 6% to 10%
   j. Platelets: 100,000 to 280,000/mm^3
   k. Reticulocytes: 3% to 6%

8. Neurological system (Refer to Section VIII-F)
9. Hepatic system
    a. Physiologic jaundice (icterus neonatorum) occurs in approximately 50% of full-term neonates and 80% of premature neonates
    b. The icteric color reflects increased serum levels of unconjugated bilirubin from increased RBC lysis, altered bilirubin conjugation, or increased bilirubin reabsorption from the gastrointestinal tract
    c. The icteris (yellow) color is not apparent until the bilirubin levels are approximately 4 to 6 mg/dL
    d. Physiologic jaundice appears after the first 24 hours of life; pathologic jaundice is evident at birth or within the first 24 hours of life (Refer to Section VIII-M-4)
    e. Unconjugated bilirubin levels seldom exceed 12 mg/dL. Peak levels occur by 3 to 5 days after delivery (full-term) and 5 to 6 days (preterm)
    f. Management requires monitoring serum bilirubin levels, maintaining hydration, providing parental emotional support, and using bilirubin lights as needed

D. **Physical characteristics of the newborn**
    1. Head
        a. Size: approximately one-fourth of his/her body size
        b. Molding: asymmetry of the skull due to overriding of cranial sutures during labor and delivery
        c. Cephalhematoma: collection of blood between a skull bone and the periosteum that does not cross suture lines
        d. Caput succedaneum: localized swelling over the presenting part that can cross suture lines
    2. Fontanels: openings at the juncture of the cranial bones
        a. The anterior fontanel is diamond-shaped; it measures 3 to 4 cm long and 2 to 3 cm wide; located at the juncture of the frontal and parietal bones; closes at approximately 18 months
        b. The posterior fontanel is triangular-shaped; it measures approximately 2 cm across; located at the juncture of the occipital and parietal bones; closes at approximately 8 to 12 weeks
        c. The fontanels should feel soft to the touch; depression of the fontanel indicates dehydration; bulging may indicate increased intracranial pressure
    3. Eyes
        a. Neonates' eyes are usually blue or gray because of scleral thinness
        b. Permanent eye color is established by 3 to 12 months of age
        c. Lacrimal glands are immature at birth, resulting in tearless crying
        d. Neonate may demonstrate transient strabismus
        e. Doll's eye phenomenom may persist for approximately 10 days
        f. Subconjunctival hemorrhages may appear from vascular tension changes during birth

4. Nose
   a. Infants are obligatory nose-breathers for the first few months of life
   b. Nasal passages must be kept clear to ensure adequate respirations
   c. Neonates instinctively sneeze to remove obstruction
5. Mouth
   a. Epstein's pearls may be found on gums and/or hard palate
   b. Scant saliva, pink lips, precocious teeth may appear
6. Ears
   a. Incurving of pinna; cartilage deposited
   b. Top of ear should be above or parallel to imaginary line from inner to outer canthus of the eye
   c. Low-set ears are associated with several syndromes, including chromosomal abnormalities
7. Neck
   a. Short and weak
   b. Deep skin folds
8. Chest
   a. Cylindrical thorax and flexible ribs are characteristic at birth
   b. Breast engorgement may occur from maternal hormones
   c. Extra nipples (supernumerary) may be located below and medially to the true nipple
9. Abdomen
   a. Abdomen is cylindrical in shape with some protrusion
   b. Scaphoid appearance indicates diaphragmatic hernia
10. Umbilical cord
    a. Cord is whitish and gelatinous with two arteries and one vein
    b. Cord begins to dry within 1 to 2 hours postdelivery
11. Genitalia
    a. Male: rugae present on scrotum; testes descended into scrotum; urinary meatus located at tip of penis (normal), on the dorsal surface (epispadius), or on the ventral surface (hypospadius)
    b. Female: labia majora covering the labia minora and clitoris; vaginal discharge from maternal hormones; hymenal tag present
12. Extremities
    a. Polydactyl: more than five digits on each extremity
    b. Syndactyl: fusing together of two or more digits
    c. Lower extremities: all newborns are bowlegged and have flat feet
13. Back
    a. Spine should be straight and flat
    b. Nevus pilosus at the base of the spine is frequently associated with spina bifida
14. Anus: patent without any fissure
15. Skin
    a. Acrocyanosis: cyanosis of the hands and feet due to adjustments to extrauterine circulation
    b. Milia: clogged sebaceous glands, usually on the nose or chin

    c. Lanugo: fine, downy hair found after 20 weeks gestation on the entire body except the palms and soles

    d. Vernix caseosa: white cheesy protective coating composed of desquamated epithelial cells and sebum

    e. Erythema neonatorum toxicum: transient, maculopapular rash

    f. Telangiectasia: flat, reddened vascular areas on the neck, upper eyelid, or upper lip

E. Sensory behaviors of the newborn

1. Tactile
   a. Sensations of pressure, pain, and touch are present at birth or soon after
   b. Lips are hypersensitive; skin on thighs, forearms, and trunk is hyposensitive
   c. Especially sensitive to being cuddled and touched
2. Olfactory
   a. Can differentiate pleasant from unpleasant odors after mucus and amniotic fluid have been cleared from nasal passages
   b. Can distinguish mother's wet breast pad from other mothers' at 1 week of age
3. Vision
   a. Can see approximately 17 to 20 cm (7″ to 8″) at birth
   b. Has immature muscle control and coordination
   c. Is sensitive to light; can track parent's eyes
   d. Prefers complex patterns in black and white
4. Auditory: can detect sounds at birth
5. Taste
   a. Taste buds developed before birth
   b. Newborn prefers sweet tastes to bitter or sour tastes

F. Reflexes in the newborn

1. Sucking: sucking motion begins when a nipple is placed in the newborn's mouth
2. Moro reflex: when neonate is lifted above the crib and then suddenly lowered, there is a symmetric extension, then abduction, of the arms and legs; the fingers will spread, forming a "C"
3. Rooting: stroking the newborn's cheek makes him/her turn his head in the direction of the stroke
4. Tonic neck (fencing position): while in the supine position with the head turned to one side, the extremities on the same side straighten while those on the opposite side flex
5. Babinski: stroking the sole of the foot on the side of the small toe makes the toes fan upward
6. Grasping: placing a finger in each of the newborn's hands will lead to his/her grasping the finger tightly enough to be pulled to a sitting position
7. Stepping: holding the newborn upright with his/her feet touching a flat surface results in dancing or stepping movements

8. Startle: a loud noise, such as a hand clap, makes the newborn abduct his/her arms with flexion of the elbows; hands stay clenched
9. Trunk incurvature: when a finger or pin is run down the newborn's back, laterally to the spine, the trunk will flex and the pelvis will swing toward the stimulated side

G. Predictable behavior during the first few hours after delivery
1. Period of reactivity: lasts approx. 30 minutes after birth; newborn is awake, active, and may demonstrate sucking reflex; has increased respiratory and heart rate. An ideal time to initiate mother-infant bonding and breastfeeding.
2. Sleep phase: lasts from several minutes to 2 to 4 hours; pulse and respiratory rate return to baseline
3. Second period of reactivity: lasts 4 to 6 hours; pulse and respiratory rate increase again

H. Gestational age assessment: see chart, p. 100 for an example of the various tools currently available for assessing gestational age

I. Nutrition in the newborn
1. Infants usually double their birthweight by 6 months of age and triple their birthweight by age one
2. Daily requirements for infants are:
   a. Calories: 95 to 145 kcal/kg
   b. Protein: 2.2 g/kg first 6 months; 2 g/kg second 6 months
   c. Fluid: 130 to 200 ml/kg
3. Newborns lose approximately 10% of birthweight within first few days of life; weight is usually regained by 10 days after delivery
4. Infants usually gain 1 oz/day for first 6 months; 0.5 oz/day in the second 6 months of life
5. Newborns are born with a 3-month store of iron if the mother had an adequate iron intake during pregnancy, according to current theory
6. The American Academy of Pediatrics recommends that formula-fed infants be given an iron supplement for the first year of life

J. Breastfeeding
1. Advantages
   a. Is economical
   b. Is readily available
   c. Promotes development of facial muscles, jaw, and teeth
   d. Aids in uterine involution
   e. Promotes transfer of maternal antibodies
   f. Enhances maternal-infant bonding

GESTATIONAL AGE ASSESSMENT (Ballard)

NAME _____ DATE/TIME OF BIRTH _____ BIRTH WEIGHT _____

HOSPITAL NO. _____ DATE/TIME OF EXAM _____ LENGTH _____

   AGE WHEN EXAMINED _____ HEAD CIRC. _____

RACE _____ SEX _____ EXAMINER _____

APGAR SCORE: 1 MINUTE _____ 5 MINUTES _____

NEUROMUSCULAR MATURITY

NEUROMUSCULAR MATURITY SIGN	SCORE						RECORD SCORE HERE
	0	1	2	3	4	5	
POSTURE							
SQUARE WINDOW (WRIST)	90°	60°	45°	30°	0°		
ARM RECOIL	180°		100°-180°	90°-100°	<90°		
POPLITEAL ANGLE	180°	160°	130°	110°	90°	<90°	
SCARF SIGN							
HEEL TO EAR							

TOTAL NEUROMUSCULAR MATURITY SCORE

PHYSICAL MATURITY

PHYSICAL MATURITY SIGN	SCORE						RECORD SCORE HERE
	0	1	2	3	4	5	
SKIN	gelatinous red, transparent	smooth pink, visible veins	superficial peeling, &/or rash few veins	cracking pale area rare veins	parchment deep cracking no vessels	leathery cracked wrinkled	
LANUGO	none	abundant	thinning	bald areas	mostly bald		
PLANTAR CREASES	no crease	faint red marks	anterior transverse crease only	creases ant. 2/3	creases cover entire sole		
BREAST	barely percept.	flat areola no bud	stippled areola, 1-2mm bud	raised areola, 3-4mm bud	full areola 5-10mm bud		
EAR	pinna flat, stays folded	sl. curved pinna; soft with slow recoil	well-curv. pinna; soft but ready recoil	formed & firm with instant recoil	thick cartilage ear stiff		
GENITALS (Male)	scrotum empty no rugae		testes descending, few rugae	testes down good rugae	testes pendulous deep rugae		
GENITALS (Female)	prominent clitoris & labia minora		majora & minora equally prominent	majora large, minora small	clitoris & minora completely covered		

Reference
Ballard JL, Novak KK, Driver M: A simplified score for assessment of fetal maturation of newly born infants. *J Pediatr* 95:769-774, 1979. Reprinted by permission of Dr Ballard and *Journal of Pediatrics.*

TOTAL PHYSICAL MATURITY SCORE

SCORE
Neuromuscular _____
Physical _____
Total _____

MATURITY RATING

TOTAL MATURITY SCORE	GESTATIONAL AGE (WEEKS)
5	26
10	28
15	30
20	32
25	34
30	36
35	38
40	40
45	42
50	44

GESTATIONAL AGE (weeks)
By dates _____
By ultrasound _____
By score _____

      g. Nutritionally superior to any other fluid
      h. Reduces incidence of allergies
      i. Reduces incidence of maternal breast cancer
  2. Disadvantages
      a. Only mother can feed infant unless milk is expressed or pumped
      b. Paternal role in infant feeding is limited
      c. Mother must monitor her diet carefully
      d. Working mother will find it difficult to maintain

K. Bottlefeeding
  1. Advantages
      a. Father and other family members can feed infant
      b. Mother is less restricted than when breastfeeding
      c. Mother can measure intake more accurately
      d. Mother can take medications without risking an effect on the newborn
      e. Infant can be fed less frequently
      f. Infant can be fed in public without embarrassment
  2. Disadvantages
      a. Costs more than breastfeeding
      b. Require greater preparation time and effort
      c. Requires cleanliness of hands, water, and equipment
      d. Requires adequate refrigeration and storage

L. General care of infant
  1. Circumcised penis
      a. Apply a thin petrolatum-saturated gauze to site to control bleeding and prevent diaper from adhering to the penis
      b. Wash penis gently with water and apply a fresh petrolatum gauze to the glans with each diaper change
      c. Apply gentle pressure with a sterile 4″ × 4″ gauze pad if bleeding occurs; notify physician if bleeding continues
      d. Observe and record first void after circumcision
  2. Cleansing and bathing
      a. First bath should be given when temperature and vital signs have stabilized
      b. Infant should be given sponge bath until the cord falls off
      c. Infant should be bathed with a mild soap, one without a hexachlorophene base
      d. Infant should be bathed prior to feeding; bathing after feeding could cause vomiting
      e. Soap may be used everywhere on the body, except on the face
      f. Each portion of the body should be washed, rinsed, and dried to minimize heat loss

3. Positioning and holding
   a. Infants are frequently positioned on side with rolled blanket supporting the back
   b. Infants can be positioned on right side after feeding to enhance gastric emptying
   c. The football hold provides adequate support for infant while freeing a maternal hand
4. Diapering
   a. Diapers should be changed before and immediately after feeding
   b. The foreskin of uncircumcised males does not retract; gentle cleaning of the penis is adequate; forceful retraction of the foreskin is not advised
   c. The vulva of a female infant should be wiped from front to back to avoid rectal contamination of the urethra or vagina
   d. Diapers should be positioned below the umbilical cord to prevent contamination
5. Temperature maintenance: normal range is 97.7° to 98.6° F. (36.5° to 37° C.)
   a. Avoid cool drafts, direct or indirect contact with cold surfaces, and exposure to wetness
   b. Take an axillary temperature every shift after temperature stabilizes
   c. Apply cap to infant's head to prevent heat loss
   d. Single- or double-wrap infant snugly
6. Pulse and respirations: after pulse and respirations stabilize, an apical pulse and respirations should be monitored every shift
7. Oral-nasal suctioning: a bulb syringe should be available to remove excessive mucus or milk from air passages promptly

M. High-risk neonate
1. Hyaline membrane disease: complex disorder manifested by signs of respiratory distress. Also referred to as Respiratory Distress Syndrome (RDS)
   a. Pathophysiology: cannot synthesize sufficient lecithin to maintain alveolar stability
   b. Clinical manifestations: tachypnea, nasal flaring, grunting, retractions, and bilateral diffuse reticulogranular density upon X-ray
   c. Assessment: the Silverman-Anderson index may be used to evaluate the respiratory status of the neonate. Grade 0 indicates no respiratory difficulty; grade 1 indicates moderate difficulty; grade 2 indicates maximum difficulty. Each of the five areas are scored 0 to 2, with a total score ranging from 0 (no respiratory difficulty) to 10 (maximal respiratory difficulty)
   d. Management: ventilatory therapy, maintenance of acid-base balance, temperature regulation, adequate nutrition, transcutaneous oxygen monitoring, and protection from infection

The Silverman-Anderson index

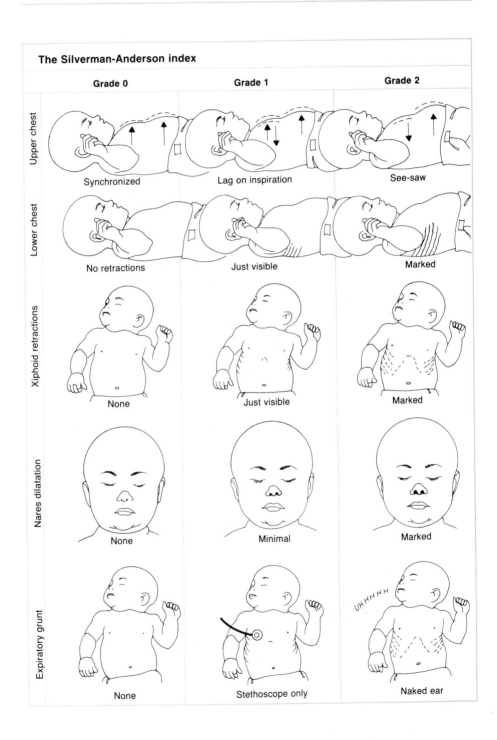

2. Meconium aspiration syndrome (MAS): aspiration of meconium into the lungs before or at delivery
   a. Pathophysiology: asphyxia in utero leads to increased fetal peristalsis, relaxation of the anal spincter and passage of meconium into the amniotic fluid, and reflex gasping of amniotic fluid into the lungs. The meconium creates a ball-valve effect, trapping air in the alveolus and preventing adequate gas exchange. Chemical pneumonitis results, causing the alveolar walls and interstitial tissues to thicken, again preventing adequate gas exchange. Cardiac efficiency can be compromised due to pulmonary hypertension.
   b. Clinical manifestations: fetal hypoxia as indicated by altered fetal activity and heart rate; meconium staining of amniotic fluid noted at time of ROM; signs of distress at delivery, such as Apgar scores below 6, pallor, cyanosis, and respiratory distress
   c. Management: immediate endotracheal suctioning of the infant at delivery, respiratory assistance via mechanical ventilation, maintenance of a neutral thermal environment, postural drainage, chest physiotherapy, and administration of antibiotics
3. Sepsis: presence of pathogenic microorganisms or their toxins in the blood or tissues
   a. Etiology: the most common causative agents are gram-negative (*Escherichia coli,* Aerobacter, Proteus, Klebsiella) and gram-positive organisms (B-hemolytic streptococci). Sepsis may be from prenatal, perinatal, or postnatal causes.
   b. Clinical manifestations: subtle, nonspecific behavioral changes (lethargy, hypotonia), temperature instability, altered feeding pattern (poor sucking, decreased intake), apnea, hyperbilirubinemia, and abdominal distention
   c. General management: collection of specimens to identify causative organisms; lumbar puncture, urine culture, skin cultures, blood cultures, gastric aspirate, and nasopharyngeal cultures
   d. Nursing management: administration of two broad-spectrum antibiotics before culture results are received, and specific antibiotic therapy after results are received; physiologic supportive care, including maintenance of a neutral thermal environment, respiratory support, evaluation of signs and symptoms of sepsis, monitoring of fluid and electrolyte balance; evaluation of metabolic disturbances; provision of cardiovascular support
4. Hyperbilirubinemia/pathologic jaundice: the bilirubin level exceeds 6 mg/dl within the first 24 hours after delivery and remains elevated beyond 7 days in a full-term neonate and 10 days in a premature neonate; it also occurs when serum bilirubin rises by more than 5 mg/dl/day and is greater than 12 mg/dl in premature or term neonates; and when the conjugated (direct) bilirubin level exceeds 1.5 to 2.0 mg/dl.

a. Pathophysiology: unconjugated bilirubin can infiltrate the nuclei of the cerebral cortex and thalamus, leading to kernicterus (an encephalopathy). Kernicterus may occur with serum bilirubin levels at or above 20 mg/dl (full-term) and at lower levels (approximately 14 mg/dl) in premature infants

b. Clinical manifestations: jaundice, elevated bilirubin levels, and hepatosplenomegaly

c. Management: treat anemia due to hemolytic disease; increase serum albumin levels; remove maternal antibodies and sensitized red blood cells via exchange transfusion and phototherapy

d. Signs of kernicterus: lethargy, decreased reflexes, seizures, opisthotonos, and high-pitched cry

e. Causes: hemolytic disease of the newborn, sepsis, impaired hepatic functioning, polycythemia, enclosed hemorrhage, hypothermia, hypoglycemia, and asphyxia neonatorum

5. Isoimmune hemolytic disease of the newborn/erythroblastosis fetalis: the breakdown of red blood cells

a. Pathophysiology: transplacental passage of maternal antibodies that cause red blood cell breakdown

b. Clinical manifestations: hemolytic anemia, hyperbilirubinemia, and jaundice

c. Management: drug therapy, family support, phototherapy, exchange transfusion, monitoring of bilirubin levels

d. ABO incompatibility can occur when fetal blood type differs from maternal blood type

e. The most common incompatibility occurs when a type O mother carries a type A or type B fetus. Type O blood contains anti-A and anti-B antibodies, which travel transplacentally to the fetus, causing jaundice and hepatosplenomegaly

f. ABO incompatibility can occur with the first pregnancy and is usually milder and of shorter duration than Rh incompatibility

g. Rh incompatibility occurs when an Rh negative mother carries a Rh positive fetus

h. A leakage of fetal Rh antigens commonly occurs during delivery, at the time of placental separation

i. Maternal antibodies are produced in response; in a subsequent pregnancy with an Rh positive fetus, maternal antibodies enter the fetal circulation transplacentally, causing erythroblastosis

j. Symptoms: hemolytic anemia, hyperbilirubinemia, jaundice, direct Coombs' test, hepatosplenomegaly

k. Prevention of Rh incompatibility: administration of Rh immune globulin (RhoGAM) within 72 hours of delivery

l. RhoGAM prevents the formation of antibodies

m. If the woman is already sensitized, RhoGAM will be of no use

    n. RhoGAM should be administered to a woman who is Rh negative and Du negative and whose newborn is Rh positive or Du positive; and to an Rh negative and Du negative woman who has had an abortion

    o. Rh sensitization can occur during pregnancy if the cellular layer separating maternal and fetal circulation is disrupted; RhoGAM can be administered at 28 weeks of gestation to decrease the incidence of maternal isoimmunizations

6. Fetal alcohol syndrome (FAS): characteristics commonly found in newborns of women who ingested varying amounts of alcohol during pregnancy

    a. Etiology: alcohol is a teratogenic substance of particular danger during critical periods of organogenesis. Alcohol interferes with the passage of amino acids across the placental barrier.

    b. Clinical manifestations: pre- and postnatal growth retardation; facial anomalies (microcephaly, microophthalmia, maxillary hypoplasia, short palpebral fissures); central nervous system dysfunction (decreased I.Q., developmental delays, neurological abnormality)

    c. Risk factors: the risk of teratogenic effects increases proportionally with increased daily alcoholic intake. No absolute safe level of alcoholic intake during pregnancy has been established. FAS does not occur only in alcoholic women; it has been detected in moderate drinkers (1 to 2 oz of absolute alcohol/day)

    d. Management: prevention through public education, careful prenatal history and teaching, identification of women at risk, referral to alcoholic treatment centers if necessary

7. Addicted newborns

    a. Clinical manifestations: high-pitched cry; jitteriness/tremors/irritability; poor feeding habits; hyperactive Moro reflex; increased tendon reflexes; frequent sneezing/yawning; poor sleeping pattern; diarrhea; vigorous sucking on hands. Manifestations of withdrawal depend on the length of maternal addiction, the drug ingested, and the time of last ingestion before delivery. Withdrawal usually occurs within 24 hours of delivery

    b. Management: tight swaddling for comfort; quiet, darkened environment; pacifier to meet sucking need (heroin withdrawal); gavage feeding if poor sucker (methadone withdrawal); maintenance of fluid and electrolyte balance; avoidance of breastfeeding; assessment for jaundice (methadone withdrawal); medication to treat withdrawal signs (paregoric and phenobarbital); promoting maternal/infant bonding

    c. Contraindications: methadone should not be given to newborns because of its addictive nature

8. Sexually transmitted diseases in the newborn: syphilis and gonorrhea

    a. Assessment: congenital syphilis is diagnosed with serologic tests at 3 to 6 months; the development of antibodies is necessary to make a diagnosis

b. Clinical manifestations of syphilis: vesicular lesions on the soles and palms; irritability; small for gestational age; failure to thrive; rhinitis; red rash around mouth and anus; copper rash on face, soles, and palms

c. Management of syphilis: penicillin therapy; isolation technique initially, followed by general care; hands covered to minimize skin trauma from scratching

d. Etiology and clinical manifestations of gonorrhea: contracted by exposure to lesion during vaginal delivery; clinically manifested as ophthalmia neonatorum (Refer to Section VIII-B-4-b)

9. Hydrocephaly: abnormal increase in the amount of cerebrospinal fluid (CSF) in the ventricles of the brain, leading to cerebral ventricle enlargement

a. Pathophysiology: alteration in either production (increased), flow (obstructed), or reabsorption of CSF

b. Clinical manifestations: head enlargement; forehead prominence; "sunset eyes"; irritability; weakness; convulsions

c. Management: skin care to prevent breakdown and infection; careful head support during handling; meeting parental emotional and learning needs; assessment of neurological status and progression of symptoms; surgical shunting to eliminate excess CSF; management of shunt and prevention of infection at site

10. Phenylketonuria: an inborn metabolic error in which there is a deficiency of phenylalanine hydroxylase, a liver enzyme essential for the conversion of phenylalanine to tyrosine

a. Pathophysiology: accumulation of phenylalanine and its abnormal metabolites in the brain can lead to mental retardation

b. Clinical manifestations: failure to thrive; vomiting; rashes; decreased pigmentation

c. Management: the blood Guthrie test, which is required by most states, should be done at least 24 hours after initiation of feedings; affected infants are placed on low-phenylalanine formula (Lofenalac) and on a continued special diet that limits phenylalanine intake. CNS damage can be minimized if treatment is initiated before 3 months of age

11. TORCH syndrome: a group of infectious diseases in the mother that can lead to serious complications in the embryo, fetus, and neonate

a. TO: toxoplasmosis; transmitted to the fetus primarily via contaminated cat litter. A therapeutic abortion is recommended if the diagnosis is made before the 20th week of gestation. Effects include increased frequency of stillbirths, neonatal deaths, severe congenital anomalies, retinochoroiditis, convulsions, and coma.

b. R: rubella; a chronic viral infection that lasts from the first trimester to months after delivery. The greatest risk occurs within the first trimester. Effects include congenital heart disease, intrauterine growth retardation (IUGR), cataracts, mental retardation, and hearing impairment. Management includes therapeutic abortion if disease occurs during the first trimester and emotional support for parents. Women of childbearing age should be tested for immunity and vaccinated if necessary.

c. C: cytomegalovirus (CMV); a member of the herpesvirus group that can be transmitted from an asymptomatic mother transplacentally to the fetus or via the cervix to the infant at delivery. CMV is the most frequent cause of viral infections in the fetus. CMV may be the most common cause of mental retardation. Effects include auditory difficulties, small for gestational age; principal sites of damage are the brain, liver, and blood; antiviral drugs cannot prevent CMV or treat the neonate.

d. H: Herpesvirus Type II; the fetus can be exposed to the herpesvirus through indirect contact with infected genitalia or via direct contact with those tissues during delivery. Affected infants may be asymptomatic for two to 12 days but then may develop jaundice, seizures, increased temperature, and characteristic vasicular lesions. A cesarean delivery can protect fetus from infection

12. Prematurity: infant delivered before the end of the 37th week of gestation
a. Etiology: (Refer to Section V-X)
b. Problems associated with prematurity: immaturity of all systems; extent depends on gestational age and level of development at time of delivery
c. Prognosis: premature infants between 28 and 37 weeks have the best chance of survival
d. Management: respiratory assessment and assistance; maintenance of fluid and electrolyte balance; prevention of infection; assessment of neurological status; maintenance of body temperature; monitoring renal function and providing emotional support to parents

13. Small for gestational age (SGA): neonate whose birthweight is at or below the 10th percentile on the Denver chart; a SGA is also referred to as small-for-dates (SFD) and Intrauterine Growth Retardation (IUGR)
a. Maternal causes of SGA: poor nutrition; advanced diabetes; PIH; smoking; over age 35; drug use
b. Placental causes of SGA: partial placental separation; malfunction
c. Fetal causes of SGA: intrauterine infection; chromosomal abnormalities; malformations
d. Problems associated with SGA: perinatal asphyxia; hypoglycemia; hypocalcemia; aspiration syndromes; increased heat loss; feeding difficulties; polycythemia

14. Large for gestational age (LGA): neonate whose birth weight is at or above the 90th percentile on the intrauterine growth chart
    a. Etiology: infant of mother with poorly controlled diabetes; multiple parity; infant with transposition of the great vessels (unknown cause); genetic predisposition
    b. Problems associated with LGA: increased rate of cesarean deliveries, birth trauma, and injury; hypoglycemia; polycythemia
15. Post-term infant: infant delivered after 42 weeks of gestation
    a. Etiology: not well understood, but associated with primigravidas, anencephalic fetus, history of postmaturity, delayed ovulation and fertilization
    c. Problems associated with postmaturity: meconium aspiration, placental insufficiency, hypoxia, hypoglycemia, polycythemia, seizures, and cold stress

Points to Remember

The neonate's cardiac and pulmonary systems must undergo major adjustments during the transition from intrauterine to extrauterine existence.

To identify deviations quickly, the nurse must be familiar with the characteristics of the normal newborn.

A newborn has four distinct needs: protection from infection and trauma; provision of nutrition, warmth, body hygiene; monitoring of physiologic adjustment; parenting.

Care of the high-risk neonate requires active support from the family.

Glossary

Conduction—loss of body heat to a solid cold object through direct contact

Convection—loss of body heat to cooler ambient air

Evaporation—loss of body heat when fluid on the body surface changes to a vapor

Neonatal period—the period between birth and the 28th day of life

Radiation—loss of body heat to a solid cold object without direct contact

Nevus pilosus ("hairy nerve")—a dermal sinus at the base of the spine; frequently associated with spina bifida.

Infertility

Learning Objectives

After studying this section, the reader should be able to:

- Describe possible male and female causes of infertility.

- List diagnostic tests commonly used to determine causes of infertility.

- Describe the couple's emotional reactions to infertility.

- Describe surgical and medical methods of treating infertility.

- Discuss possible options for the infertile couple.

IX. Infertility

A. **Infertility: the inability to conceive after 1 year of consistent attempts without the use of contraceptives**
   1. Types of infertility
      a. Primary infertility: neither the man nor woman has caused impregnation or been pregnant
      b. Secondary infertility: the woman cannot conceive or sustain a pregnancy after an initial pregnancy
      c. Sterility: presence of an absolute factor that prevents pregnancy (male or female factors)
   2. Incidence: infertility affects approximately 15% to 20% of couples in the United States
   3. Possible female factors causing infertility
      a. Endocrine disorders
      b. Obstructed genital tract
      c. Anatomical abnormalities (cervical, tubal, vaginal, uterine, or ovarian)
      d. Emotional disorder
      e. Preexisting medical conditions
      f. Severe nutritional deficit
   4. Possible male factors causing infertility
      a. Obstructed genital tract
      b. Spermatozoan difficulties (decreased sperm count, decreased motility, malformed sperm)
      c. Abnormal genital tract secretions
      d. Coital difficulties: cannot deposit sperm at the cervix; may be linked to obesity
      e. Testicular abnormalities due to illness, cryptorchidism, trauma, or irradiation
   5. Diagnostic measures: female
      a. Menstrual, medical, fertility, sexual, surgical, occupational history
      b. Physical examination
      c. Review of personal habits, including medications, smoking, alcohol, exercise, weight history, use of douches or vaginal deodorants
      d. Laboratory examinations: complete blood count, sedimentation rate, serology, urinalysis, thyroid function tests, glucose tolerance tests
      e. Cervical mucosal tests
      f. Postcoital sperm analysis to assess sperm mobility and morphology
      g. Hysterosalpingography to assess tubular patency
      h. Culdoscopy to assess tubular function
      i. Laparoscopy to view pelvic organs directly
      j. Monitoring of basal body temperature
   6. Diagnostic measures: male
      a. Medical, surgical, urologic, sexual, occupational, surgical history
      b. Physical examination

    c. Review of personal habits, including medications, smoking, clothing, alcohol, bathing

    d. Laboratory examinations, such as sperm analysis, complete blood count, urinalysis, sedimentation rate

7. Emotional reactions to infertility

    a. The couple may demonstrate behaviors associated with loss: surprise, denial, anger, bargaining, depression, and acceptance

    b. Infertility leads to decreased self-esteem, feelings of inadequacy, loss of control over life, and loss of acceptance by society

    c. Medical investigations into infertility lead to embarrassment, decreased privacy and disruption of normal, spontaneous marital relations

    d. The infertile couple who ultimately conceives may exhibit the normal ambivalence associated with pregnancy (Refer to Section IV-C-1)

8. Management of infertility: treatment modes are numerous and depend on the causative factor

    a. Surgical management: correction of anatomical defects and removal of obstructions in the reproductive tract

    b. Medications used when infertility is due to anovulation: Clomid when ovulation is inhibited by hypothalamic suppression; Bromocriptine when ovulation is inhibited by increased prolactin levels; Synthroid when ovulation is inhibited due to hypothyroidism; Pergonal when ovulation is inhibited by hypogonadotropic amenorrhea

    c. Medications used when infertility is due to hormonal disorders: conjugated estrogen and medroxyprogesterone in hypoestrogenic states; hydroxyprogesterone in luteal phase defects

    d. Medications used with the male: Delatestryl and Depotestosterone to stimulate virilization; Pregnyl to virilize a hypogonadotropic male and to restore spermatogenesis; Pergonal to aid hCG to complete spermatogenesis

9. Options for the infertile couple: artificial insemination, in vitro fertilization, adoption, and surrogate mothering

    a. The number of infants available for adoption has severely decreased because of decreased social stigma of out-of-wedlock pregnancies

    b. There are many legal and ethical ramifications associated with artificial insemination, in vitro fertilization, and surrogate mothering

Points to Remember

Infertility can be viewed as a major life crisis.

Infertility can decrease self-esteem and strain marital relations.

The nurse must be sensitive to the invasion of privacy that accompanies infertility testing.

Infertility can occur even after the woman has already given birth (secondary infertility).

Glossary

Artificial insemination—the mechanical depositing of donor or partner's sperm at the cervical os

Basal body temperature (BBT)—the temperature when body metabolism is at its lowest; a way to determine whether ovulation has occurred. The BBT is usually below 98° F. (36° C.) before ovulation and above 98° F. postovulation

Cryptorchidism—undescended testes

In vitro fertilization—fertilization of an ovum outside the female body with replantation of blastocyte into the woman

Surrogate mothering—conceiving and carrying a pregnancy to term with the expectation of turning the newborn over to contracting, adoptive parents

Index

Notes

Notes

Notes

Notes

Notes

Notes

Notes

Notes

Notes

Notes

Notes